The Road to Mana

Finding Healing, Happiness, and
Power on the Way to Life

Kimberly R. Kelley, MD, MBA

The Road to Mana
Finding Healing, Happiness, and Power on the Way to Life

Disclaimer

The information, ideas, and techniques in this book are not medical advice or treatment, but rather knowledge intended to assist the reader. It is the responsibility of the reader to seek treatment for any medical, mental, or emotional conditions that might warrant professional care.

All characters and events depicted in this book are entirely fictitious. Any similarity to actual events or persons, living or dead, is purely coincidental.

THE HOLY BIBLE, NEW INTERNATIONAL VERSION®, NIV® Copyright © 1973, 1978, 1984, 2011 by Biblica, Inc.® Used by permission. All rights reserved worldwide.

Scripture taken from the New King James Version®. Copyright © 1982 by Thomas Nelson. Used by permission. All rights reserved.

ISBN: 978-1-946978-84-4

Dedication

To the men and women who serve and sacrifice self for country—those who serve humankind and those who serve for our well-being. May you enjoy peace and good health on this road of life.

To the soldiers who have made a difference in my life: Charles and Dorothy Kelley, Irving "Will" Harper IV, and Kim M. Bradford. Sometimes the greatest battles are fought not on foreign soil but on familiar soul. May you find peace in the valley.

To my children, Will, Ari, and Aaron, my raison d'être. May you always listen and follow the soft voice within.

Contents

Preface

There is no greater agony than bearing
an untold story inside you.

—Maya Angelou

This is the story of five people who come together for one week, looking for peace and a way to deal with the chaos of life. Anxiety, depression, burnout, compassion fatigue, and moral injury laced with regret have dimmed their prospects of living full and happy lives. They have heard that Sister, a well-known woman of healing, offers weeklong retreats at her home in a Hawaiian paradise and might have what they need to help them find their way back.

Lew—A veteran, husband, and father, Lew has been diagnosed with posttraumatic stress disorder (PTSD); he is having trouble keeping it together. His wife, Lois, has given him an ultimatum. The drinking and anger are just too much for her. He is bright, self-medicates daily, and walks for hours when the demons come. Lew confides in his friend, Pat, as a last resort. He and Lew served together during Afghanistan and Iraq deployments as sergeants. Pat had been on this retreat several years earlier, so he knows the work that Sister could do. Lew is the life of the party and loves to laugh and joke. It is all a façade to hide his sad heart. He is a soldiers' man, a protector of men and women. He protects everyone and loves them all, except for himself. His heart aches, and he cannot find peace. "Lew, trust me, she can turn your life around," Pat had said. "I don't know what your plan is, but God does; there is no shortcut, it's hard work, but you just have to do it." Lew jumps out of the truck at the gate on Mana Road as Pat points in the direction of the way to Sister's house.

Sara—Though happily married to her stay-at-home husband with whom she has two children, primary care physician Sara is becoming increasingly cynical, depressed, anxious, and moody. On paper, Sara's life is a dream—picture-perfect with hubby, kids, career, nice home in a gated community, a dog, and a cat. Sara's friend, Vonna, and she have mirrored lives—both married with children and careers in the medical profession. As they chat in the doctors' lounge, Vonna finds Sara is out of touch. Sara has just returned from a Disney vacation with her family, but still seems despondent and worn. Sara realizes she has given so much to everyone, especially her patients (despite receiving negative satisfaction scores), leaving nothing for herself; she feels empty. "Sara, you need to get away," advises Vonna. "Really, Vonna, I just got back!" Sara replies. "Yes, but that doesn't count; the kids and Isaac were there too." Vonna offers to give Sara a week of her vacation. After some initial resistance, Sara warms to the opportunity to visit an alternative healing retreat for rejuvenation that she's always wanted to attend. "My in-laws are coming that week; I prefer to be working," Vonna snickers. Sara knows Vonna is right. If she continues this way, she will be of no benefit to herself, her family, or her patients. At the airport, Sara kisses the kids and wipes her tears as her hubby drops her off. "Go, honey, we'll be fine. By the time you get back, the baby will be potty-trained," he grins and winks.

Uncle Ira—A farmer who struggled with cocaine addiction when he got out of the service soon after the Vietnam War, Ira came to Hawaii, just wanting to get away from it all. He married a local girl, and her love for him, along with the joy of raising their children, straightened his path and gave meaning to his life. Now in his seventies, Ira had been a successful coffee farmer on the Big Island. His wife passed away from breast cancer two years ago. And then, two months ago, the hostile takeover of his farm by his sons, who sold out to a genetically modified organism (GMO) firm, left him broken in spirit and in heart, and lost once again. He lives a four-hour drive from Sister's place, on the other side of the island, but has heard of Sister and her legendary healing. He wants to live again and to stop hurting. He drives his truck up the narrow, muddy Mana Road to the gate that leads to Sister's place with no expectations and little hope. It's just something to do, one last try before quitting life. He is searching for meaning, value, and redemption.

Nora—An ambitious, energetic woman at the top of her business class, on the executive track, and accepted at the University of Pennsylvania Wharton business school, Nora fell in love and married her classmate. Four years and three children later, dreams deferred, she is a frustrated housewife watching her husband travel to establish himself in the industry. She loves her husband and her children but feels undervalued in her relationship and underachieving in the mundane world of motherhood. She is searching for fulfillment and gratitude for motherhood. She needs to change the direction of her life and desires secret permission to move forward. Her mother-in-law senses her frustration and offers support, while Nora's husband is gone for yet another three-week business trip. She shows Nora a brochure of Sister's retreat and offers to keep the children. Nora jumps at the opportunity for a getaway—anywhere!

Reiko—The only child of a real-estate mogul, who wants to turn over the reins of his empire to her and the man he has arranged for her to marry, Reiko is uncertain about her future. Yet, she doesn't want to disappoint her father. Biracial, Reiko drifts between both cultures, Japanese and African-American, showing no dominant traits of either. Her personality is a blend of fine arts and mathematics. She has not embraced either culture but is looking for her own identity. She has come to Hawaii with friends to get away and sort it out. While hiking with her friends at the Hawai'i Volcanoes National Park, she notices a flyer for a retreat posted in the lobby of the ranger's office. Looking for self-discovery and acceptance, she would love to be a bird and just fly away from her troubles. Instead, Reiko finds herself hiking up the winding Mana Road to Sister's place, hoping for inspiration, insight, and direction.

Each chapter represents a healing practice as revealed through the essence of one of these retreat participants. Sister helps these individuals unpack some of the unconscious stories they have been carrying and reframe them in truth, using a new lens and a different perspective. She provides tools for the wayfarers to carry home in the form of an enlightened understanding of nutrition, movement, mindfulness, meditation, massage, and yoga. These simple practices, based on ancient traditions of the mind-body-spirit connection, are the first steps toward healing on the road to mana.

With Gratitude

My Parents

Charles and Dorothy Kelley, I was born to you, so you could provide me with the environment to accomplish my mission on earth. You have been the perfect parents to nurture my education and foster my appreciation of the simple things that only Mother Nature can offer.

My Children

Will, Ari, and Aaron, you are my pride and joy—this one is for you. I am so proud and excited for each of you. Will, for you who are my constant motivation, especially for your brave heart. Ari (Willie), my doll baby and her prince, for your awesomeness in raising a family, and showing that fairy tales do come true. Aaron, wise old actor, for your patience with my parenting. Charmaine, second daughter (niece), for your devotion and smiles.

My Grandchildren

Kayla (Lil Princess), Grant, Isaac, Solomon, and those twinkling stars whom we have yet to meet, I hope you realize your fullest potential and know that all things are possible—as above, so below—always choose to be happy!

My Family

Sisters, Karen, Tamara, Lucinda, and Kathleen, and brother, Clarence (Carla), for playing your roles well as characters in this game of life. Thank you, Cindy and Karen, for your kindness.

My Love

For your constant devotion, support, belief, love, companionship, and patience.

My Inner Self

For your patience, love, and persistent soft voice; you are the raindrop on the rock.

My Friends

Kim, for feeding me when I was hungry; for listening, believing, loving, and caring when the road was dark; for your counseling expertise with a Southern flair; for your editorial support of the characters; your input has been invaluable. You are amazing! **Sabrina**, for your love, support, and devotion during the middle passage; you have been a true soul sister. **Revonna**, for your friendship through the lean years and for pushing me professionally beyond my comfort zone for one last hoorah. **Jennifer**, for listening without opinion. **Kay**, for school days. **Mayumi**, for your introduction to the way. **Medical School Musketeers**- Bill and Petty for your belief, support and laughter when I first came to CSU.

Pat and **Lois**, for your wisdom, guidance, friendship, honesty, and support, and editing from PEMBA and beyond—*the business mind* and *the whisperer*; your absolute love, support, and direction will always be remembered.

Bob and **Pauly,** for your warmth without questions; for opening your home when I needed a place to rest; and for your hospitality, advice, and safe haven. You provided the space for me to reflect, grow, and write.

Koa, the dog, for taking me out in the evening for walks under the moon and for laughing at me.

My Swim Pod

Pauly, the zen swimmer who taught me to listen to my breath, even underwater. **Nancy,** for your soft love and gentle wisdom. **Ellie,** for your loving kind friendship and always willingness to swim the lagoons. **Sang** and **Su,** for the fun and laughter in and out of the water. **Lysa,** my dolphin buddie, for saying yes when we saw them at Kealakekua bay.

Core Wellness Hawaii

The originals, **Kim, Sheila,** and **Dana,** for believing in and supporting me, and for your incredible work ethic in the dream. Kim (counselor, for your insight and originality); Sheila (yogi, for your balance and kind spirit); Dana (for your amazing counseling creativity).

Richard, for your enduring love and friendship.

Matthew, for your encouragement and kindness @mile 15 and beyond.

Torri and **Uvo** for your support of my work when it was in utero.

Henry Hao for your artistry in painting the Mana Road.

My Teammates - Panthers, Buckeyes, Marauders, Raiders, Army buddies, PEMBA colleagues, and Navy shipmates for your support both spoken and unspoken in this game of life

Kathleen Shewman for bringing my thoughts alive on paper.

Best Seller Publishing for providing the platform.

Introduction

Two roads diverged in a wood, and I—
I took the one less traveled by,
And that has made all the difference.

—Robert Frost

Mana Road, situated near the magnificent mountain of Mauna Kea in Hawaii, is a 40-mile, narrow, dirt road that winds by sweeping vistas of windblown forests, koa woodlands, and rolling green pastures. It is a place where the distant ocean seems to kiss the clouds. The beauty of this road calls you to adventure, to explore the farms and wildflowers, horse stables and woods; yet the captivating power of her beauty fully settles into your heart only after you have journeyed deeper into her wilderness.

We all have stories that have shaped our lives. Difficult life events sometimes disrupt our understanding of the world around us. Our personal responses to these events influence our ability to glean wisdom, knowledge, and awareness. This can hinder our ability to move forward, choosing a healthy direction and quality relationships.

Mana is also a road that can lead to self-discovery. This forgotten path might be a lonely path, but one that can be all the more rewarding and ripe for exploration and self-revelation. We find ourselves on this road, looking for answers to life's most intimate questions. The path we traveled to get to this road is unique, but the quest for truth is universal.

Welcome to the road to mana. May you find peace and joy as you walk.

Ha'ina mai ka puana—Let the story be told.

Hotep—peace

Chapter One

Awareness

The first step toward change is awareness.
The second step is acceptance.

—Nathaniel Branden

The rich aroma of freshly brewed Kona coffee wafts through open rooms filled with morning light. It draws the guests to the kitchen, a bright welcoming space filled with delicate sweet scents of mango and pineapple. As the newly arrived participants trickle in from their rooms to start their week, the sounds of quiet pervade the air and engage their senses—the gentle rustling of wind through trees, the jaunty chirping of birds celebrating a new day.

The clucking of hens adds its own kind of satisfying rhythm to the mix. The only bit of possible discord breaking through is the intermittent jarring crows of a rooster. No voices, no background music. Simply the incredible beauty of nature, manifest in the stunning views through the open windows.

The crisp, balmy air drifting through the spacious, sunlit rooms is cool and sweet. The vista to the south lures the eye along the horizon, where sky meets ocean in subtle shifts of shading, blue on blue. Palm trees and pine trees seem magical, giving an impression more of Narnia than of Hawaii. Off in the distance, the white-capped summit of Mauna Kea can be seen.

The house sits atop a small hill just off a road. The view permits seeing any person approach, long before such a traveler would notice the structure. The well-manicured lawn in front of the house is bordered on the right by the garden. Strutting around the yard is the now-famous rooster, and the hens and chicks are pecking along the other side of the porch. Kiwi, the cat, is busy scurrying around in the bushes. On the porch, a black Labrador named Koa is stretched out resting in a lazy sprawl.

Four of the five guests who arrived the prior evening mill around the kitchen and dining area. The simple, sunny space has a calming effect, bringing them into this day with a quietude that none of them is ready to spoil with small talk. Three of them are wandering around the clean, well-kept rooms, appreciating the sparse furniture crafted in the old Hawaiian style. They inspect the artwork hanging on the walls, paintings—friends of their host and scenery—extending from the dining area into the hallways. One piece has ensnared their attention, and three strangers gather to study it. Names form some type of picture, but their curiosity does not solve the mystery.

Their host, whom each met briefly upon arrival the previous day, is nowhere to be seen. The fourth guest, a woman, remained in the kitchen, leaning against the counter. She turns and notices a blackboard on the wall behind her. A note says, *Help yourself to fresh coffee, tea, and fruit. Please meet me in the garden in thirty minutes.* Sara picks up the coffee pot and shows it to the others, pointing at the message with a tight smile. They abandon the artwork and join her. She returns the pot to the warmer and steps back.

There is a stirring behind them, and all heads turn to see a tall, attractive man in his early thirties bound into the room. He seems full of energy, as a morning person would be, yet he exudes an air of grumpiness that would announce a night owl forced from bed too soon. He is wearing a red shirt and jeans—and sunglasses. He stands there with his gaze roaming the room, then he takes a deep breath and lets out a loud sigh, saying: "Hmm, smells like home."

A few smiles, but no one speaks. He takes a pineapple from the fruit array on the counter. Expertly cutting into it, he pulls out a glistening chunk on the tip of the knife and pops it into his mouth. He closes his eyes, enjoying the sweet moment. He prepares the rest of it, pours himself a large cup of coffee, and then, noticing the woman standing a few feet away, he grabs another cup and holds it out to her.

"Hi, I'm Lew. You want some coffee?"

Eyeing the cup warily, she answers, "No, thanks. I'm Sara. I'm more of a tea drinker." She says this with a slight emphasis on the last two words, as if being a tea drinker carries some significance.

Lew drops the hand holding the proffered cup and steps back for a better view of Sara, an average-looking woman with brown hair touching her shoulders, wearing a simple floral blouse and brown slacks. She appears a little older than Lew, and tired. Really tired. He nods and turns, pointing toward the other counter holding the teapot. He cannot help but roll his eyes once his head is angled away from her view.

Sara, who had noticed the tea service as soon as she entered the room, now takes this moment to move toward it. She slips around Lew with awkward maneuvers to avoid contact. She gives him a quick smile, glancing up, as he stares down the more than half a foot difference in their heights. He does not return the smile.

An older gentleman, about seventy or so, comes up behind Lew and stretches out his hand for the extra cup. "Man, I'd love a cup of Kona."

Lew turns toward him, handing him the cup. He notices the man's sturdy hands, with permanent ground-in dirt around the nails. "I'm Lew, uncle. Nice to meet you."

The man responds cheerfully, "Good to meet you, Lew. My name is Ira." He adds with a wink, "Call me Uncle Ira." He fills his cup and wanders out to the porch to pet Koa.

Lew carries his coffee and a bowl of pineapple chunks to the table and settles in to eat. Sara brings her tea to the table and takes a satisfying sip. She glances at Lew, who is fully focused on his breakfast, his head bent toward the bowl.

Taking a measured inhalation, Sara says, "So, Lew, what do you do?" Her clear expectation is that he will provide a brief description of how he makes his living, and then inquire after her life's work. Lew looks up, a little surprised, and sits back against his chair. Taking his coffee cup in hand, he imbibes a long swig, then places it back on the table, before replying, "I'm not much of a morning person, Sara. If you don't mind, I'd just as soon skip the small talk for now. No offense."

Sara drinks another sip and seems a little flustered. "Oh, sure. I'm sorry. No offense. None at all. I'm kind of worn out from my flight, so I understand. All the way from Knoxville, Tennessee; can you believe it? I'd never thought about traveling to Hawaii until, well, just before I flew here for this retreat." After a quiet moment, she adds, "I think I'd also like some fruit, actually." She moves toward the large fruit bowl on the counter and grabs a mango.

Lew watches as she dispassionately, almost violently, slices the soft fruit with a knife, the fruit's raw, severed flesh wet with juice. He looks away. With a soft shake of his head, he turns his attention back to his breakfast.

Over the next few minutes, the guests wander outside to the garden, as instructed. They settle on log stumps set in a ring in a grassy area near the garden entrance.

Soon they hear the mellow sounds of deep humming, and Sister emerges from the garden all of a sudden, as if she had been standing there, camouflaged, all along. Her smile is all they notice on first sight. It occupies her entire face, radiating warmth and sparkling with the pleasure of being alive. She is a beautiful, ageless woman with lovely bronze skin that shows only the slightest of wrinkles. As she pulls off her gardening hat, her soft, brown curls flow around her face and deepen the color of her earthy eyes. Her sarong, a becoming garment of green and yellow, with bold accents of bright red and deep purple, flows around her tall, strong body in the light breeze.

"Aloha!" she calls out, lingering over the long vowel. In a low, soothing voice, she adds, "Welcome to you all. I am so delighted you have come."

The stunned guests notice their host is barefoot. She is holding a huge basket of fruits, herbs, and vegetables she has picked—mangoes, apples, tomatoes, green onions, ginger, basil, cilantro, avocados—and eggs. Beautiful speckled eggs are visible, resting on a nest of spinach. She holds up the basket with a grin, and says, "Lunch." Placing it on the ground, she spreads her arms wide. No one has moved, and they clearly have no idea what to expect.

When they met Sister the prior day, she was congenial, but more restrained, as she showed them to their rooms. Sister looks around the circle, as if taking a moment for herself to absorb their presence. Then she steps up to Lew. She is nearly as tall as he is, a woman of regal bearing. She takes his hand as if to shake it, but leans in and envelops him in a hug, pressing her open palms into his back.

This sudden move surprises them all, especially Lew. Nonetheless, he adjusts and politely accepts this gesture. They are all taken aback when she does not release him after a few seconds, the commonly acceptable time for a hug between strangers. She holds on for at least twelve seconds, about ten more than any of them think appropriate. Sara squirms a little, but stands her ground, waiting for the next step in this questionable enterprise. The others smile awkwardly and stare away from Lew and Sister.

Finally, Sister releases him and steps back, still holding his arms in her sturdy, slender hands, as she stares intently into his eyes. After a moment, Lew reaches up and removes his sunglasses with one hand, revealing a bruised eye—dark, and surely painful. Sister continues to gaze into his face, then nods, and moves on to Uncle Ira. She works her way around the group, giving everyone equal time. No one gets away with less than the full twelve seconds.

During all that, Sara, who is the last to receive her hug, has had time to prepare herself. She accepts the embrace with good grace, giving Sister tiny pats on her back every few seconds, as if to signal: All is well, you can stop now, to no effect. Sister does not deprive Sara of one second. But the hard part is not the hug. It is the searching, loving gaze into her eyes afterward. Sara finds it difficult to maintain eye contact through this. It leaves her with a strange feeling, not knowing if she was intruded upon or given more comfort than she has felt in a long time.

At last, Sister reenters their band. She regards them, not as a group, but one-to-one as she moves her eyes around the circle. Slowly, she says, "I am so delighted you have found your way here. I hope you will always call it home. You have journeyed so far to come here, to tell your story. What you encounter here this week might make you laugh, might make you cry. But more important, I hope it will make you grow."

Sister asks the group to connect pinky with thumb, person-to-person, around their circle. Stretching out both hands, she grabs Lew and Sara's hands on either side of her and slides each into position, locking her pinky with Sara's thumb and her thumb around Lew's pinky. The others quickly follow suit, and they find they have formed a tight, interlocking band with these new people in their lives.

Sister gives this a long moment, and then says, "Become aware of your hands, of the tight bond we are forming in this circle. We form this circle because the circle represents us. This represents our wishing well through this week. I wish you well. I wish you wellness through this week. I call this the DANA well—deserving, desiring, and needing answers. I want you to come to understand that this is our sacred space, our sacred place, and we want to, in essence, honor it, if you will."

Everyone remains still. Waiting. Then, Sister continues, "In the mornings, I want us each to put something into the well. After we have gone through each day, I want us to be able to take something out of the well."

Sister inhales deeply and nods toward the opening formed in the center by the joining of their hands. "I'll go first. I want to pour into our well, hope, and love. I want you to—I want us to—grow. I want us to become part of one another. I want us to be respectful of one another. I want us to be authentic and transparent."

Beaming, she says, "I hope that you will smile and dance, as if you were a child. Your basic needs will be met this week. You will have food, and shelter, and companionship. I hope the real growth will come in finding the other pieces of your life that will satisfy the hunger of your heart and quench the thirst of your soul."

Sister grows more solemn. "This is a sacred area of trust we are creating. We will not all agree on all that is said. But I ask you to be respectful as a listener and respectful as a speaker. I trust you will be truthful and transparent in your interactions. This is a sanctuary for you. Can each of you verbalize your agreement with an affirmative yes?"

Sister fixes her eyes on each face, as each affirms agreement with a yes. She turns her head to Lew and says, "Lew, what would you like to pour into the well?"

Lew pauses, then says, "Well, I want to pour in anger. I get tired of losing my cool at the wrong moments, and then regretting it."

Sister nods and turns to Sara. "Sara?"

Sara is suspended on a deep breath for a moment. Her eyes remain fixed on the ground. "I want to put in acceptance and confidence. I want acceptance for who I am, not what I do."

Uncle Ira takes his turn. "I want to put in understanding. I want to understand why my family treated me the way they did."

Sister nods at Uncle Ira and turns to Nora. "Nora?"

Nora glances around, not stopping for eye contact. "I want to put in energy and hope." She smiles, adding, "I hope I get something out."

Reiko is next. She says simply, "I want to put in fear. I want to receive courage to do what I want with my life."

After Reiko speaks, Sister says, "I want to tell you a story from the Hawaiian tradition that was told to me when I first arrived. Let's walk in the garden first." She smiles and says, "Please remove your shoes."

They hesitate but comply.

"It's okay. The ground is soft. Feel the grass and earth under your feet. Come, come into the garden. The garden is where we grow." She waves her hand to draw them to follow her into the garden. They step tentatively but follow her through the entry into the lush foliage. "Welcome to my office," she says with a jubilant laugh.

She gives them a tour of the garden. The air is suffused with an array of delightful scents, some floral, some savory. Stopping in a grassy clearing in the center, she sits on the ground, motioning for them to join her in a ring.

"When I first arrived in this beautiful place, I was told this story." Although her eyes are full of energy, Sister speaks slowly in a low voice, inviting listeners.

> "The *kūpuna*, our wise elders of Hawaiian ways, told me this tale of a bowl of light from the Hawaiian tradition. Each child is born with a bowl of perfect light. A child will grow in strength and health and can do anything, as long as he tends his light. The child can swim with the sharks, soar with the eagles, know and understand all things. If, however, the child becomes envious or jealous, he drops a stone into the bowl, and some of the light goes out. Light and stone cannot hold the same space. If there is hatred, envy, or unkindness—these are stones that are placed in the bowl. The light will go out, and, eventually, the person will become stone.

"A stone does not grow. Nor does it move. At any time, if the person wearies of being a stone, all he needs to do is turn the bowl upside down. The stones will fall out, and the light will grow once more.

"Huli huli, turn upside down." Sister gestures, as if she is turning a bowl upside down.

"The bowl of light represents each of us and our true heart—light and love. When we are conscious and respectful of this light, we are living in our highest state of being. We are mindful and aware, on our true path of freedom. The stones in the bowl represent pain and suffering that occur when we resist life, instead of trusting life. If our bowl of light becomes stones, we feel disconnected from our source of love. To turn over our bowl of light and dump our stones is like starting life again.

"Now, it is not possible to eliminate our past or deny it. What we can do is return light to our bowl, so that the memories of our wounds no longer affect us negatively. We are able to see life differently, with a fresh perspective, through a new lens. We will come back to this."

Sister leans back and says, "And now, you may remain in the garden or wander around. We will share lunch in the dining room in one hour." She stands, pushing up on strong legs in a graceful movement. Taking hold of her floppy hat and the harvest basket, Sister walks toward the kitchen door to go prepare a meal, leaving each of her five guests blinking in wonder at the world in which they now find themselves—a world of color, of life, and of strange, new possibilities.

People take different roads seeking fulfillment and happiness. Just because they're not on your road doesn't mean they've gotten lost.

—Dalai Lama XIV

Chapter Two

Movement

The essence of bravery is being
without self-deception.

—Pema Chödrön

Lew

Simple, fresh, and delicious is the food Sister prepares and places before the small group, who accept it with gratitude. Papaya; wild green salad with ginger, watercress, cilantro, and sesame seed oil; macadamia nut butter with honey; banana on cranberry bread; and plenty of lemon water, tea, and coffee. A light meal, but they all eat plenty of what is there. They chat and enjoy one another's small talk, under the spell of the good food. Nora laughs, "Yummy, this is the best peanut butter and banana I've ever had!"

Teaming up to clean the kitchen afterward, though still a little awkward with one another, they make a good effort at coordinating the tasks and get them done in a short time. Sister is heading toward the door with a water flask from the fridge in her hand, having put on her slippers and some jeans. She faces them where they stand, hanging up dish towels and giving the table a last wipe.

"Hey, we're going to go on a short hike, and then, we're going horseback riding." She beams. "So, grab your flask from the counter, and let's head out. We're going right now."

Sister bounds out through the door, and then stops, holding it open with one hand to look back at them. "Any questions? Everybody good?"

Each of them looks at her and glances at the others, responding with affirmative shakes of their heads. So, Sister nods and takes off through the door, then heads around the left side of the house. As she starts through the field toward the trail, Koa jumps up from her spot by the back door, where she'd hung out during the meal, and trots after Sister. Her tail is wagging hard; she likes the company and she likes a journey.

All quickly follow Sister out the door, walking at a good pace, but not quickly enough for Lew. He breaks into a little trot and catches up with Sister. Sister points Lew toward the trailhead and says, "Hey, Lew, I know you have energy, just follow the trail. It'll take you up and down hills, and through a few little pastures, and then a wooded area. Some of it's overgrown, but don't worry about it, just stay on the trail. Then, you'll see a road, and right across from the road, there's a barn. Before you get there, though, on this side of the road, you will see a large tree. You'll know it. So that's where I'll meet up with you."

"No worries. Got it," Lew responds, taking off through the field at a brisk jog.

Sister reaches down to pet Koa and urges her on to catch up with Lew. Koa takes off after Lew and bounds up beside him, glad to accompany someone who is moving at a faster pace. Sister then drops back a little, slowing for the rest of the crew, who are taking their time and enjoying the lush, sweet day.

Lew is fast on the trail, and Koa is matching his pace, even bounding ahead at times, and then winding back, adding many more steps to the hike than necessary. But she's full of joy and pleasure. And it also makes Lew realize how good this walking is making him feel. It's hot now, but the breeze is cool against the sweat on his skin and fragrant as it blows through the foliage.

It has been awhile since he's hiked like this, moving through open countryside, feeling his muscles support his bouncing stride. When he was a platoon leader, he would move like this most of the time, sometimes with a good deal more caution. Leading soldiers, he had to keep them on track and keep them safe. Lew is a natural leader. His soldiers respected him.

Despite the good feelings and the positive energy from being in nature, after thirty minutes or so, Lew's body is feeling heavy, unduly anchored to the ground. No alcohol in a few days, no pot, and it's not like he planned it that way. The food and now the hike are helping, but he has a ways to go in lifting this sluggishness, this mental fog.

For a brief moment, his mind drifts back to a vivid picture of his time as a scout in the Army. The face of one of his buddies comes up in his mind like a full moon. The four of them had been through the mill together. Hot as hell, through never-ending days in the desert during that long deployment. Then freezing his butt off on patrol at night, damn scary. Day after day like that. What had he been thinking? He wasn't. Just a crazy high school kid anxious to get on with his life. Then, everything changed one day and set in motion the direction of his life in response to that one day. It was the day the war on terrorism began.

They dismissed class for the high school kids to go home to be with their families. Lew ran all the way and came bounding in the back door, letting the screen door slam hard, but Mama didn't say a word.

She and Papa were transfixed in front of the TV; the second plane had just hit one of the Twin Towers. They sat there all day like that, the three of them. Isaiah, his younger brother, wandered in later, after the bus dropped him at home, but he didn't seem to grasp it. Lew's gut felt twisted and empty. And he knew he wanted to serve his country, like his grandparents.

After graduation, going off to Hawaii for school was exciting. He studied for the ministry. Having been raised by two devout Christians, it seemed a natural thing to do. But he also joined the reserves. And boy, the recruiter got him good. Promised him $5,000 as a bonus to sign up for the infantry. And lucky him, another $5,000 to boot, if he signed on as a scout. And $10,000, to a nineteen-year-old, might as well have been a million. It felt like that to him. He'd scored well on his exams and could have had an administrative job. But not him. "What the hell was I thinking?" Lew ponders, the words slipping aloud through his lips. "That's not worth a hill of beans to me now."

As he approaches the wooded area with Koa, he stops in place on the trail and looks up toward the sun. He is really feeling the heat. The trail has narrowed through an endless section of brush, and the tips of the weeds are sliding along his arms, leaving scratch marks. His mind drifts back to Ohio: working in the fields that summer after Papa got him that gosh-awful job detasseling corn. He made a ton of money in two-and-a-half months but was that job a bear! His arms were all torn up, and his hands were splintered and callused.

"Man, that was nothing compared to what I had to do on my first deployment," he mutters.

His mind drifts once more. He is back in the desert. Waiting, always waiting. Almost unbearable, the long hours, and missing his parents and the hometown he'd been so anxious to get out of. Koa barks and brings Lew's attention back to the trail. He emerges from the tight wrap of bushes, where the path opens to a wide hill in the distance. Without a thought, he takes off bounding toward and then up the hill with renewed energy. Koa flies after him and lets out a few sharp barks, scaring some birds that take off.

Flashing back, Lew hears the loud *pop-pop-pop* sounds around him— gunfire—and he drops into a crouch as he keeps running. He hears the helicopter over his head, circling, the engine pounding in his ears, driving the hard *chop-chop-chop* sounds of the spinning blades, and he sees the fire—bright-orange flames spreading suddenly overhead— and he thinks, *Fuck! This ain't no video game!* He drops to his knees. The island heat beats down on him, as he realizes he is in Hawaii.

Breathing hard, he stays put on his knees, facing the high grasses on the hillside. That was the day, damn it. He remembers doing what he had to—pure instinct. He'd been well-trained as a sharpshooter, and he had a knack. When Papa taught him to hunt with a gun, he'd never pictured this. He hadn't been the kind of kid to play war games or dream about battles. Under pressure, he'd just gone deep and focused on what he needed to do. He'd achieved cover, and he got his soldiers theirs. He got them out of this little predicament. He had several kills that day. He took them into his awareness, and then set them aside. Just information.

But when he got back to base, he was a big hero, and everyone was congratulating him. That is what the Army trained him for in the first place. What does a boy who studied for the ministry do with all that? So, he stuffed it inside and accepted their praise and their drinks. Lots of it.

Lew looks up to the sky and stands. He hears someone calling his name. He turns back toward the trail, and, in the distance, he sees the group walking with Sister. He waves to them and sees them return the greeting. He stretches and puts his arms overhead to absorb the full feeling of this moment. He takes a deep breath and closes his eyes, grateful for this moment of life. Here in Hawaii. On this mountain. Halfway up the hill.

He sees Reiko nearby approaching. She hails him cheerfully. A young woman, fit, in her early twenties. Clearly an athletic woman, and she had mentioned at lunch that she enjoys hiking. Then Lew notices farther down the trail, Uncle Ira is behind Reiko, but ahead of the others and about halfway up the steep, grassy hill; he seems a bit out of wind. Lew rushes back to meet him and give him a hand. They take their time getting to the top, with Lew's encouragement. It helps, and when they are at the top, Lew looks back and sees the others closing in. He waves again, and then, turns and runs down the other side of the hill, with childlike abandon.

As he runs, a child's face appears before him. He knows it is in his mind's eye, but it almost seems disembodied, floating in front of him. Lew lets out a choking sound and slows as he reaches the bottom. He keeps walking, picking up the trail. But he is back in the desert, in his Humvee, dirty; he's on patrol, and as he drives, fine dust clouds rise up around him. He sees his little friend. He gave him candy that first time they'd met, as he asked him questions in his broken Arabic. Cute little guy, maybe twelve. Open and smart, not timid. Reminds him of Isaiah. Hard not to like him.

"Hey, Haji," he calls out in Arabic, "you know anything?"

"No, no," Haji replies in his broken English. "Tomorrow, tomorrow. I don't know."

On patrol the next day with his buddies, Lew sees another boy, older than Haji, flagging them down, looking frantic. He's fairly sure it's Haji's brother. This boy's English isn't as good as Haji's, and Lew isn't sure what he wants. But he keeps pointing and yelling, "There! There!" So, they put him in the vehicle and take off to where he directs. And there, inside an abandoned building, just inside the door, is Haji. Lying on a pile of debris, his throat cut, his mangled body's blood still freshly flowing.

Lew feels his throat and chest fill with a hot liquid as heavy as lead, and he looks at his patrol mates, his buddies, who grab his arms and pull him back to the Humvee. And back to the unit they went, and then that night, back to the village. No clear picture ever comes to his mind of what took place, or how they got there. But he remembers shooting. And darkness. He doesn't know who cut the throat of that innocent child. But he remembers shooting. All of them. They were shooting.

Lew stops again. He can see the road ahead. He feels like he might throw up and bends over to let the feeling wash over him. He looks up and sees a building for the first time since he left Sister's house. A barn. It could be a building from the village where he was just running in stealth, hiding, shooting. But he knows better. He pictures just then, not Isaiah, but his own little boy, Solomon. Kid's not even three. What kind of father does he have? What can I do for him? He stands there a moment and takes some of the advice he'd recently given to Uncle Ira; deeply breathing, he takes some time to get himself back on an even keel.

Lew hears his name and looks back to see Reiko coming along at a good clip, calling out, "Lew! Lew! Lew!"

Lew points to the barn, now in sight, and waves her along, calling out, "Hurry up, we're almost there." But then he turns to his right, and there is the tree. He feels it in his gut at first sight. This is the spot.

# # #

A young handler comes out of the barn and waves at Reiko and Lew, who are waiting under the huge, convoluted-looking tree. "Hey, whenever you guys are ready, let us know. Horses are all hitched up and ready to go." They watch Koa running around, wildly wagging her tail and barking at the horses. Not aggressively. The man lets them know Koa and the horses are old buddies, and she's singing out her greetings.

Soon after, Sister and the others show up, and they all settle under the designated tree to talk. She asks, "So, how many of you have ridden horses?"

Lew pipes up, "In elementary school, for a while. At church camp."

Nora says, "Yeah, I was in 4-H and rode a bit in high school."

Sister says, "Great. So, some have, and others have not. It might be a little frightening for you, but it's a great activity. I think you'll enjoy it. So, if you'll trust me, I've matched horses to each of you based on your personalities."

She looks up and opens her arms upward, palms up, fingers pointing toward the winding, knotted branches of the bizarre tree rising above them. "But first, let's rest a bit under this banyan tree. Look at the branches, how they intertwine and form stronger, larger branches. Our lives are like that, intertwined. The banyan is not native to Hawaii but thrives here. It begins its life in the crevices of a host tree, and, as it grows, its roots drip downward, looking like a fall of hair, hanging from the branches to reach the ground. Are the roots coming out of the earth or falling into the ground? Eventually, these twisting threads, these roots, crowd and engulf the host. This sacred tree represents eternal expansion. Legend has it that God Krishna often rested in its branches. And that it was under the bodhi tree, which is in the same family as the banyan tree, where Buddha sat and received enlightenment."

Sara chimes in, a little excited, her words tumbling out, "You know, I've seen these trees before. I traveled to India, when I was a medical student. So, this is not the first time I've sat under a banyan." She smiles and looks around the group. "They're actually fig trees, and some of them grow to enormous size. I recall they have many ecological benefits, and there have been studies done that support the many long-standing medicinal uses of the banyan."

As she speaks, Lew abruptly stands, glaring at Sara for seconds that seem longer, then he turns and walks away. She stops speaking mid-sentence, and they all watch Lew walk off without a word. Sara says, "Well, I really don't recall the details just now." And with a tight smile, she falls silent. Reiko says, her voice only slightly audible, "He's rude."

Ira shakes his head, as he watches Lew walk away, but he smiles slightly. Sister has risen now, and Ira gets up and holds out a hand to Sara, who takes it with only a slight hesitation. Before they leave the banyan, Sister stops to scoop some sap from the tree and offers it to Nora. "May I?" Nora nods in the affirmative, and Sister rubs it gently on a red spot on her leg. "Should be completely gone by the time we get back," and she adds with a wink, "unless you fall again."

Lew has wandered ahead of the group across the road toward the horses. Walking up to one, he gently strokes her neck, and tries to dispel the agitation that woman has raised in him. "What a know-it-all bitch," he mutters softly.

Two handlers come out of the barn and tutor everyone on the basics to control the movements of the horses. And then, Sister says, "You know, with the horses being matched to you, they'll understand you some and feed off your energy. The trail can be narrow, and there are some hills, but these horses have walked this trail many times. They'll keep you safe. Be at one with the horse; try to get into the groove as you're riding on the horse, and just go with it."

They all mount, Nora and Lew managing on their own, Ira and Reiko needing a little more assistance from the handlers, who hold their horses' heads to encourage them to stand quietly. Sara stands back, observing the others, before taking hold of the saddle and attempting to get her left foot into the stirrup. But her horse pulls away, and she seems a little embarrassed left standing there trying to regain her footing. Sister takes hold of her horse's reins and leans her forehead against the horse's head, and after a moment or two the horse relaxes. One of the handlers brings over a stepstool and helps Sara mount. Sister mounts her own horse then and takes up a spot next to Sara to ride along as her companion.

Another of the handlers takes up a position next to Nora, as it is clear she is the most comfortable, and gives her some instructions as they head out. Then he falls back and rides next to Reiko who is third in line, after Lew. They head out, with horses leading the way. Occasionally, Sara's horse—older, slower, stubborn—stops to eat shrubs. Sister is able to intervene and help her through it. She reminds her to relax and fall into sync with the horse's movements—to trust her a little, be one with her. Sara nods a little stiffly in agreement, wanting to be a good student.

The ride seems hypnotic. The scents of the grasses, trees, potent flowers, and air rise up around them, as the intense warmth of the mid-day sun penetrates their skin, creating a drowsy sensation, exaggerated by the rocking movements of the horses.

Arriving at a waterfall, they rest, letting the horses drink their fill. They lay around and splash a bit under the tumble of the water, enjoying the icy feel. Refreshed, they all mount up and head back. It is a short ride, and for Sara, somewhat intimidating, though she does not acknowledge it. But everyone feels happy, and a little excited, once they are back. They are feeling grounded and satisfied. They head to Sister's place together, chatting a little as they walk. Even Lew hangs in there with the group.

# # #

A fine day; full of a pleasing dinner—Okinawa potatoes, roasted veggies, peppers, onions and herbs, salad, watermelon, and quinoa bread—the group is sitting back on the stumps near the garden. They find themselves spellbound by the sun moving down through the sky, saturating it with hues of gold, pink, and purple. Soon the world is a pitch-black expanse, punctuated only by a massive display of stars, rarely seen by modern-world people. The only other visible light is a dim glow from the kitchen and the campfire.

Sister's voice is soft and unexpected as she says, "Look at the stars. Shooting stars! Twinkling stars! You know, our ancestors are these stars. And these stars are here to guide us. Breathe in deeply and slowly. Take in the beauty of this moment. Take in what you experienced today."

Their eyes are adjusting to the low light. Sister looks around and asks, "So how was your hike today? And your ride with the horses? Tell us something about that." She looks in Uncle Ira's direction, and says, "So, Uncle, how was it for you?"

Ira puts down the stick he was using to write his name in the dirt. "Well," he replies, "I noticed a lot of fruit trees. I had no idea there were so many fruit trees out this way. I stopped a lot to look at them, and I ate some mangoes and some mountain apples. Here," he says. He pulls several pieces of fruit from his baggy pants pockets and passes them around. "I bought some apples and strawberry guava to share. Between the dinner and the fruits, I'm feeling good right now, full and happy." He pats his stomach softly.

"Anything else?" Sister asks. Ira shakes his head no. "Good, good," Sister replies. "What about you, Lew?"

Lew says in a quiet voice, "It felt so good to move. To run without caring. To just let my body go full steam ahead, and move, and run sometimes, whenever I felt that urge. Can't always do that at home. No open spaces. I was able to do that today. I let out a lot of pent-up stuff." He recalls Sister discreetly handing him a packet of herbs after dinner with instructions to brew some tea, which he did. He is feeling somewhat better, a little more clear-headed and relaxed. "Thank you, Sister," he adds, without specifying for what.

"You're welcome, Lew," she says, before turning to Nora. "What about you, Nora? How was your day?"

"I was at peace. I still am. Sitting up on that horse was wonderful, like drifting off, taking a hot bath. I was just living in the moment. At times, I even closed my eyes and let the horse be my guide, while I breathed and, well, just breathed. I felt so alive. So aware."

Sister lightly pats Nora's arm, and then turns to Sara. "Sara, anything you want to share about your day?"

After a pause, Sara speaks up, "Well, I enjoyed the walk. It was good to be in nature and just take it in, not thinking about staying on a schedule. And about that ride, I'm not sure what to think. I'm glad I did it. I tried hard, but I've never been on a horse. I enjoyed the feel of movements of my horse's muscles under me, and her warm body was so soft. Overall, I think the horse was not too pleased with me, but I enjoyed stroking her soft hair, and I think she liked that too." She laughs a little. "But once I got off, and knew I had done it successfully, I felt really good. A sense of accomplishment." She waits a moment and then, says, "Thank you, Sister, for riding with me. It really helped me stay with it."

"I enjoyed it too, Sara," Sister says softly. "Reiko, your thoughts?"

"It has been a long day, and I am tired, but also so energized. I love feeling my body working, the muscles moving and strengthening, and all that hard work and sweat being constantly balanced with the beauty of this place. I felt a sense of joy and balance. Whether I was off on my own or walking and talking with all of you. I felt solid. Balanced."

Sister looks around at them and sees how exhausted they are from this full day of moving their bodies in nature. *Between the hike, the horseback ride, and the high-altitude with a lower oxygen content, which they are not accustomed to, they will sleep well,* thinks Sister.

After a few minutes of quiet, Sister says, "I think you all had a good day. Some growth. Awareness of living in the moment in this wondrous life. Being grateful for the simple, natural things in life can heal you. We walked, and then rode. Walking, running—those things will heal you. And you can run to something." She looks at Lew. "Or you can run *away* from something." She looks over at Reiko. "Running to *self*, to find self. I hope each of you will find yourself here."

Sister takes a long soft breath and says, "This is the beginning of your healing—getting to know your authentic and true self. Becoming aware of that which surrounds you. Each day is a gift for each of you to open. A present from the universe. I am giving you this box made of koa wood to symbolically place your gifts into daily. This box will be a constant reminder of the gifts you receive. Every day is a present, a surprise to you from the universe. Unpacking daily with gratitude is the best way to learn to appreciate the gifts that the universe has for you. If you find something you enjoy, then put it in the box. This will be your treasure chest of magical gems to draw from in times of need— be it emotional, physical, or spiritual.

"As you reflect, write, or meditate on your activities from the day, my hope is that you transform these life lessons into tools you can use to excavate your true self. As we move forward, most times we have to look back. Go back and take a different path. The box is a tangible way in which to hold your experiences. It is your well from which you will draw upon. It is your tool box to build your dreams. The box is your opportunity to receive the gifts of the universe."

Sister walks up to each of them and places a small box in each upturned palm.

"Consider beginning your day by opening your box, your present, your gift from the universe. Start your day with what you put in the day before. Let this be your foundation.

"This koa wood you are holding is legendary in Hawaii. It is native and highly revered—sacred. It has deep rich colors and a varied grain pattern. It was *kapu* (forbidden) for anyone to possess other than the monarchs and *ali'I* (royalty class). The inner beauty and inner strength in each of you is just as beautiful as this wood. Your spirit, your soul, your grain, your stripes, your heritage, and your culture is reflected in your thoughts and how you appear today. Some of you are more aware of and knowledgeable about your past. Others of you are just starting to open these channels.

"*Koa* means *warrior*. It is used for weapons and canoes. The bowls (*umeke*) you eat from and the gardening tools (*niho' oki*) are all made of koa wood. You will touch it and receive its warrior mana. It is plentiful in this area. These stumps you sit upon are koa wood from fallen trees. It will energize you in the mornings; it will give you power during the days; it will provide you solace in the evenings during our circle time."

Sister stands and holds out her hands on each side, making it clear they will now reopen their wishing well. They move toward her and Nora and Uncle Ira take Sister's hands, locking fingers to thumbs with her and the person next to each of them. "Reiko," Sister says softly, "tell us what you are taking from our well this evening."

"I saw this beautiful butterfly today as we walked in the meadow." Reiko speaks with an elated voice. "I was thinking of the brilliance of Mother Nature and how magnificent the colors are—blue, black, white, and yellow. I know that butterflies mean change and good luck."

Sister says, "That's right, Reiko. Butterflies represent transition, renewal, and change."

Reiko adds, "I take out transformation! I could have followed that butterfly to the mountain and back. It seemed to dance and to play with me. I feel light as a feather."

"Sara?" Sister asks.

"I just enjoyed the wispy clouds and the kiss of the mountain breeze on my face. I felt like running free through the prairie." Lew glances over at Sara, wondering if she is trying to impress someone with her poetic phrases. "I take out freedom!" Sara announces.

Nora is next, and she says without prompting, "I was so busy looking at the mountain, relishing it in the moment. It was so majestic and seemed to draw me to it. I tripped over a fallen branch, and that grounded me for sure." She giggles as she touches her bruised knee. She cannot see it in this light, but it isn't sore or swollen. Actually, it feels fine.

Sister looks at the knee without breaking from the circle, and says, "Is it better?"

Nora replies, "Yes. It is." She sounds a little amazed. Sister smiles. "I take fun out of the well! I was tired on the trail, but it was invigorating and fun. I fell, but I had fun!"

Lew speaks up after a quiet moment. "I saw two trees on the trail while riding the horse. The horse had strength. Even though he was bigger and stronger than me, he allowed me to control and steer him. I felt powerful and strong. Still, the horse knew the trail, and I could rely on him to not let me take him off of it. The two trees reminded me of my little brother and me. They were together but leaning from the harsh winds. That's what I think he and I are up against—some challenges. I take out power."

Uncle Ira says, "Sister, I live on the other side of the island, but I had forgotten how rich the soil is over here. I haven't been to this area in years. Just too busy. I picked *lilikoi*. My horse and I had our fill of mountain apples and strawberry guava. My knees hurt a little. Not from the hike, but from my horse bouncing around." He laughs and continues, "The *aina*, the land, is good here. I want to take out soil."

Sister says simply, "I take out the pleasure of experiencing this day with all of you and taking part in your healing and growth.

"Thank you for your deposits to the well. There are no right or wrong answers, so no need to judge. These are gifts we share with the universe. The universe graciously accepts your gifts and will respond in kind.

"Now, as you go to your rooms tonight, take a moment to reflect on your day. Remember your feelings. Remember what captured your imagination. What made you smile or laugh? What made you feel sad or unhappy? Did you feel as if you were a child again?

"Think of the butterflies that captured Reiko's imagination, arrayed in colors of life—blue, black, white, or yellow. Some days are dark, some blue, like blue Mondays. But the butterfly still flutters happily around, dancing in the wind. Butterflies come from change. From metamorphosis—one state to another. There is resistance. Struggle. But like the butterfly, we too can change—transform.

"This is the beginning of your awareness. As you prepare to retire for the day, give your attention to the stars. They will guide you on your journey. We will talk more about this later. You have had a long day and need to rest. You are all welcome to stay awhile and sit out here on the stumps and take in your day or just stargaze." She adds with a smile, and a broad curving motion of her wrist, as if turning over an invisible bowl, "huli huli!" They all return the gesture and smiling say, "huli huli!"

Sister stands to leave, and as she passes Lew, she hands him another small sachet of herbs. She speaks to him in a whisper, bending near his face. She peers deeply into his eyes, reading his energy with concern. "Drink this tonight, Lew. You will feel better in the morning." She places her hands on his shoulders with a slight pressure, "And when you are ready to share, I will be here to listen." She stands and walks toward the kitchen door.

"See you all in the morning." She waves and disappears into the house.

# # #

After Sister has been gone for a few minutes, Lew rises and goes into the kitchen to make the herbal tea. He sips it and lets the soothing sensations sink into his body. He carries the cup to his room, as he thinks about his day. He felt wonderful during and after the horseback ride. He loves to hike, but the ride was unexpected. He turns out the light and feels like king of the hill.

His mind drifts back to combat days when he was the fastest up and down the hills. He could easily sprint up and down, get a soldier out of danger with his lightning speed and strength. They called him "Flash," and he smiles a bit at the memory. Bad knees and all. Somehow, it just didn't seem to matter back then. He reflects how he feels free and unbound. Wide open spaces, ironically, make him feel safe. They hold his spirit and protect him. He slips off to sleep with a smile on his face.

# # #

Reiko snuggles into bed and closes her eyes in the dark. Behind her eyelids are colors, though. She sees a lustrous butterfly. Its colors do not have distinct lines of separation, but merge. She sees them melding into a new blue, a beautiful turquoise blue—unlike any other. She thinks of her own desires—she longs to feel loved, cherished by someone who really knows her, understands her. A sense of hopefulness fills her center. A smile lights her face as she falls asleep.

# # #

Sara sits out in the dark a little while longer than the others. Only Ira remains when she finally gets up and heads to her room. Sitting at the tiny table next to the open window, she thinks about what Sister said about the butterflies. Her world at the hospital feels limited to black and white only. How can she find a way to be with her patients in a compassionate way? How can she find a way to give solace and peace while delivering bad news?

She is so distant and stiff with them, when she knows they need more from her. Just the facts. That's what she relies on to make it work. Just give them the facts. She sees their faces and she feels for them but doesn't know what to do with that. "I can get you some pastoral support, if you need to share," she hears herself saying in a tight little voice, not sure whether to place her hand on an arm, or just stay wrapped in her own personal space.

She hates to deliver news about the dreaded "C" word, cancer. She was trained to not give in, to not cry. Not show her feelings, certainly not at the bedside. She longs to make contact, to comfort, but cannot bring herself to do more than say, "I'm so sorry." Even then, she finds herself avoiding their eyes. It makes her feel so powerless, inept. She can't imagine telling any of this to the group. Will she need to do that? She writes her thoughts in her journal, then places it under her pillow, before falling asleep.

# # #

Nora, lying in her bed, drifts back to an evening in her childhood. She was reminded of that time today. Running in the fields chasing butterflies with her friends. They were at the church picnic. Gosh, she couldn't have been more than six years old. Good times. She reaches down and runs her fingers over the bruised knee. No pain. She pulls it out from under the blanket and looks at it. No bruise. Smiling, she turns off the light and falls asleep, satisfied to let her body rest after a long, energetic day that has left her utterly relaxed.

#   #   #

Ira remains on a stump, watching the stars, watching the moon. He has a lot to think about. Farming is in his blood, and he loves that. Everywhere he sees the richness of the soil, the abundance and beauty of the plants, the essence of nourishment it represents. He has to do things differently, if he is to farm again. Maybe, this change the butterfly represents will be good. But now, it is time to rest.

The wound is the place where the Light enters you.

—Rumi

Movement - Recap

*Without mental health there can
be no true physical health.*

—Dr. Brock Chisholm, World Health Organization

Lew—Physically fit, but emotionally unhealthy.

Sister's Solution—Nonpharmacologic treatments: exercise, focused physical activities (horseback riding, canoeing, hiking), herbal support, and plant-based medicine.

Exercise—Positive effect on depression, anxiety, stress, and PTSD. It can predict morbidity and mortality by affecting weight loss and glucose control. Exercise promotes bone health and mental health and increases immunologic factors. Insufficient exercise results in increased rates of cardiovascular disease and all-cause mortality. Not only can a physically active lifestyle reduce mortality and prevent many chronic diseases, such as hypertension, diabetes, stroke, and cancer, it can promote healthy cognitive and psychosocial function.

Chapter Three

Nutrition

*Raise your words, not your voice. It is rain
that grows flowers, not thunder.*

—Rumi

Uncle Ira

Lew and Uncle Ira wander together through the extensive grounds of Sister's garden mid-morning on the second day of retreat, both feeling satisfied and at ease. Lew finds Ira's energy appealing. A solid man, not that tall, but well-built from a life of hard work. Ira's muscles have that hard, sinewy look of men who make their livings outdoors, engaged in manual work, just doing what needs to be done for long hours. And he does it cheerfully. He has not soured on a life like that—he's thrived on it. And yet, he is sad. Ira has a stillness about him, and Lew senses more, despite Ira's willingness to engage in easy banter and his readiness to smile.

Ira stops as they wander into a small grove of trees. He cups one of the odd little fruits on a tree in his sturdy hand, and again Lew notices the callused fingers and the ground-in dark rings around his nails. A lifetime of work has colored his hands with hues of the earth.

And then, Papa's face pops into Lew's inner vision, and he realizes how he always thought of Papa in that same vein. Simply bound in a visceral way to the land. Papa's hands look as rough and darkened with dirt as Ira's.

"Hey, Lew," Ira calls back to him. "See this?" He holds up the fruit tucked among the leaves, without removing it from its tree. It is unlike any fruit Lew has seen before. An uneven yellowish-white surface with a bumpy texture of dark pebbly points poking through its skin, it looks as if it's full of seeds anxious to burst through the skin.

"These are ripe, my friend. Here, take a sniff." Lew bends toward the fruit in Ira's hand and inhales the cheesy odor. Lew wrinkles his nose and steps back.

"Was that a trick, Uncle?" Lew laughs. "What's up with that? I've smelled better stinky cheese in my life."

Ira laughs and said, "No trick. Just want to show you something special. The *noni* tree. This stuff is really good for what ails you. I'm not surprised Sister has so many of these on her land. They're great for healing. Well-known in the islands for uses in plant medicine. Ancient medicine, powerful. Just about anything you can think of, this stuff will help."

Lew runs his thumb over the fruit's surface and smiles. "Good to know, Uncle." He adds with interest in a tone of respect, "You know a lot about things like that, I'll bet."

"Oh, yeah. Well, I've been at this for a while." Ira bends and touches a patch of loose soil; then he scoops up some in one hand, letting the dark moist granules slip through his fingers as he sifts them with a deft movement of his thumb.

"Had a lot of responsibilities, you know. Three kids and a wife. A great wife." His voice goes a little soft on that last comment, and he nods to himself. "When I came home from Nam in 1971, I scrambled around for a while trying to get a handle on things. My life." He grins to himself at the memory, then shakes his head, as if he can't believe it. He glances up at Lew, who stands quite a bit taller than he does, and notes Lew's attention fixed on him.

"Tell you what, Lew," he says, "back then, when I was your age, my friend, I was young, and I was dumb." He says each word slowly and pauses, before adding, "And just trying to get me some." He gives Lew a quick shove on the shoulder and grins, and Lew cracks up.

"Good one, Uncle," Lew laughs. And again, Papa's broad face appears in Lew's mind. Papa is actually old enough to be Lew's grandpa. A good man, not biologically related to Lew, but he raised him, along with his wife, whom Lew calls Mama, even now as an adult, and Lew couldn't feel closer to any two people. Except his brother, of course. Papa always had a special kinship with Lew; he would take the opportunity, once Lew became a teenager, to tell him a "dirty" joke now and then, when he thought Mama was out of earshot. And he also tried to teach him to farm. But Lew wasn't inclined to it.

Ira points out several other plants, mentioning possible medicinal qualities and how they taste when edible. He mentions having grown taro (*kalo*), for years on his farm. He seems to take some pride in that but does not go into detail. But coffee was the big crop. He keeps checking the soil as they walk.

"This is rich land. Good soil. You know, anything can grow here." He looks up at Lew, and Lew feels deeply reassured by him. He seems to have a handle on things. Knowledge, rootedness. Lew wonders why he is here for the retreat.

"Hey, Uncle, how'd you end up here? You seem to know an awful lot about many things," Lew ventures. Ira remains quiet, and Lew wonders whether Uncle feels he is prying.

But then Ira replies, "Eh, well, you know, Lew. I'm like everybody else. I'm kind of searching too. Just because I'm old, doesn't mean I know everything. I just don't want to be an old fool," he adds, with a forced guffaw that reveals a slight wrench in his voice. Then he goes on, "So I know a lot about the land." He shrugs, "I know a lot about life."

Ira turns to face Lew and says, "What I know about is the land. I know how to respect the land. I know how to honor the land." He falls quiet, and Lew does not rush to fill the silence, as he absorbs Ira's meaning.

"Lew, the land is like a woman. Because that is what the land is. We call it *aina*. She feeds us. She nourishes us. In India, you know, the people honor and respect the cow, because the cow nourishes and feeds the people. She gives them sustenance. She gives them milk. Indigenous Americans respected and honored the land too, knowing that she sustains and nourishes in all seasons. In ancient Egypt, the goddess Hathor was identified with the image of a cow, providing nourishment for the people."

Uncle Ira laughs after a moment and says, "Yeah, man, you can't live without a good woman in your life."

A gentle breeze is blowing, and the air is so fresh out in these far reaches of Sister's garden. Lew stretches and sucks in a deep lungful. He loves being outdoors. Lew feels a sudden longing for the simplicity and joy of the life this good man must have led all these years. He too might have been able to have that had he stayed in Ohio, not gone off to the military, but farmed as Papa hoped he would, or if he had worked toward the ministry. Maybe he could have been the one with the timeless wisdom to offer someone at this point, or at least building a life that would eventually take him there.

Uncle Ira looks up at Lew suddenly and says, "You know, Lew, I've got sons your age. And I had a farm. And my boys sold it right out from under me to one of those GMO companies. The company leaders gave each of my sons a brand-new truck, and they told them they would give them $100,000 each, if they would sign off on letting them come in and plant their GMO seeds. Around here, in Hawaii, that kind of money is a lot for young folks. You flash that kind of dough in front of youngsters who don't have a lot of cash, and they end up making bad choices. So, anyway, now they've got the GMO crop in, corn of all things, and it interferes with our native seeds, and that's just not right."

Ira is shaking a little as he speaks. "I never saw it coming, but they voted me out. My own flesh and blood. I know their mother would be turning over in her grave if she knew about this, what her own boys have done. Damn, the deceit, the deception of those two." He takes a deep sigh, and says, "I don't know what I did wrong. Why did they turn on me like that? Guess I'm just an old mule, and they outgrew any use of me they might have had."

Ira continues after a moment, "Well, when I found out what they did, I got in my truck and just drove on down the road. I ended up driving myself to the hospital, because I got an awful chest pain. They did all these fancy tests on me—said my heart was just fine. One of the doctors said maybe I had a chest spasm or something. But my old heart was right as rain, yes, sir." Uncle Ira clutched at his chest suddenly, and said, "You know, from time to time, Lew, my heart does hurt, but it's just heartburn, that's all it is. I guess I just have to live with it."

Lew mumbles, "Heartburn, heartache, it's probably all the same." He really doesn't know what to say to Ira, and then, he remembers it is about time to get back. His stomach is rumbling, reminding him they now have about fifteen minutes to hightail it back to the house for their late morning lunch. He says, "Hey, Uncle, we ought to get back now. Don't know about you, but I could use some grub."

# # #

They enjoy an early lunch of papaya salad, vegetable soup, bread, and a variety of ripe fruits, along with small talk, which Ira mostly listens to rather than joins. But it is a pleasure, and he pays close attention to what each of them says and laughs along when the others are laughing. Nothing gets too somber over a good meal.

Ira is coming to appreciate their little group in the time they have been together. He thinks, "So much can come clear about a person in a short time, and when that time is concentrated through mutual activity and focus, you can learn a great deal—if you pay attention. Not so different than it is with plants, which spring from all kinds of soil. Actually, it has been far easier to understand plants than people. Sure, I've been getting better at it in recent years, but, boy, do I ever regret how long it took me to see the people in my life with any clarity."

His daughter's image comes to mind. An educated woman, as he had wanted, and a happy wife also. He had not really given much thought to what would make her happy. Just that he had to get his little girl into college, and then, she would marry.

Ira has not seen Sabrina since she came home for the funeral when his Dottie passed. Before that, she'd been gone so long, living with her husband in Georgia on their farm. He imagines her walking the rows of soy, a baby in her belly, her second. She bends now and then to examine the tiny leaves sprouting from thin, translucent stems, smiling and consulting with her man. She looks radiant.

So much he had held back from her all those years, all the times she had wanted to learn about the workings of their family farm. She was a smart, loving girl. But he could only see Willie and Chuck as his farming legacy. She grew strong anyway, watering her own thirsty stem, and achieved her dreams, studying agriculture and marrying a farmer.

"Dad," she'd said, distraught at seeing him so lost, sad, and angry, on top of his grief over losing her mom, "come live with me. We could use your help for sure on the farm, and you could get away from all these constant reminders of what used to be."

Ira felt sad whenever he thought of his sons, and how they had let him down. And he felt sad when he thought of his only daughter, and how he had let her down. He counted himself lucky she did not appear to hold it against him.

Ira ponders what he put into the well that morning—*betrayal*. The sadness from profound betrayal encompasses him like an invisible, wet cape, weighing him down wherever he goes, robbing him of the lightness he used to feel in his life. He used to wake early every day and get up without hesitation, ready for the blessings, or the hardships, of the day. Either way, he felt ready and light, able to rise to the occasion. Now, things feel more like effort.

He recalls yesterday's hike when he slowed on that high grassy hill on the trail, and how Lew came bounding down the hill, young as he is, and assisted him to the top. It made him feel a longing that he could not pinpoint right away. He realizes Lew reminds him so much of his older son, both of them actually, and he wished in his heart that one of them would do something like that for their dad. It also reminded him that, strong as he has been all his life, he is getting old. He sighs loudly. When Nora, who is sitting next to him, turns her head to see if he is okay, he smiles a little sheepishly.

# # #

The group emerges from the woods onto the beach at the bay. Sister has assured everyone it will be a short canoe ride to the tiny uninhabited island that is the target of their quest today. But all they can see is the wide, open sea, lapping toward them a little too vigorously for them to grasp the wisdom of setting out on it in anything less than a good-sized motorboat. Yet, there is the skimpy six-person canoe in front of them. They will all be expected to sit in it on the open water, and row with some degree of coordination against the waves. They cannot even discern out on the horizon the proposed island destination.

It is a beautiful place Sister has brought them to, but no one seems to be taking it in, other than Ira, who cannot help but notice such things. He feels strengthened by these surroundings. He is not put off by the idea of the canoe trip. He is strong enough, even at his age, to contribute to the rowing, and he has been out on the ocean before in similar craft. He can see the trepidation of some of the others. Sara hasn't said she can't swim, but it is written on her face. And Lew seems concerned also. Not fear. Something else.

Sister leads the way to the canoe, and says, "Let's sit for a few minutes before getting underway."

They all sit on the beach and remain quiet. Sister urges them to a silence by taking a deep breath and raising her arms gently overhead, then lowering them again in a graceful gesture, palms down. Ira thinks, *huli huli*, as he pictures the stones drop from his bowl. They all complete the gesture after her and take a few silent breaths. Sister says nothing, and they sit quietly, waiting, listening to the roll of the ocean, cocooned in their cove by dense foliage and by the bay, as each wave hits the sand and rolls within a few feet of their circle.

In the silence, Ira recalls walking the unpaved road up the hill to Sister's house on the afternoon he'd arrived. Breathtaking views surrounded him, as he'd basked in the crisp mountain air, and the beauty of the fields of wildflowers and trees displaced his sadness for the time, filling him with joy. He'd heard of Sister, and after the blows in life he'd been dealt, he was delighted to come to her to learn. Arriving near the house, he was blocked by a brook too wide to jump, running along a wooden and stone fence. He obeyed the sign, removing his shoes to cross the stream, and, on the other side, he put on one of the pairs of slippers left there. It had pleased him.

Sister's serene voice ends the silence.

"Let's talk story with an Aesop's tale. An old man on the point of death summoned his sons around him to give them some parting advice. He ordered his servants to bring in a bundle of sticks. He said to his eldest son, 'Break it.' The son strained and strained, but with all his efforts, he was unable to break the bundle. The other sons tried, but none of them was successful. 'Untie the bundle,' said the father, 'and each one of you take a stick.' When they had done so, he called out to them, 'Now break it.' And each stick was easily broken. 'You see my meaning,' said the father. 'Union gives strength.'

Ira mumbles to himself, "I should have read this story every night to my boys." He pictures their faces the night of the vote, filled with greed and betrayal. It makes his throat feel tight and lumpy, and he forces himself back to the immediacy of Sister's words.

Sister says, "We will all work together to get to our destination. It's not far. We have to work as a team, or we won't get there. The island is not occupied. We'll be wearing vests in the canoe, which is a solid craft that will serve us well. "

Sister stands and reaches into the boat, pulling out a vest. She demonstrates putting it on correctly. Then, she motions for them to do the same. There is some hesitation, but finally Ira and Reiko get up and pull out vests to put on, and Nora follows. Sara hangs back, and Sister nods her head to encourage her.

Lew pulls out a vest and holds it in one hand for a moment before saying, "Sister, you know, I've kayaked, and I think I would do a lot better with my own boat. Any chance of me using a kayak?" There is the slightest hint of irritability in his voice.

Sister looks at him with a smile and a tiny shrug, as she pointedly looks around for a nonexistent kayak. Lew takes a breath and starts putting on the vest.

Sister says, "There are six seats in this canoe, so we will each take one. Ira, I think you would do well to sit at the head of our canoe, and Lew, I think you would be best just ahead of me near the back." She looks at Reiko, and says kindly, "Reiko, you can sit in the center. Nora and Sara, either remaining seat would be fine."

# # #

Sara falls, attempting to disembark on Flat Rock Island. Sister had given an explicit explanation of how to row, focusing on the critical elements of working the motions in tandem; otherwise, they could not move through the water effectively. Sara had started to feel somewhat competent, contributing what she could, keeping in sync with the others.

But standing, as the canoe rocks a little at the landing, half in and out of the water, is nerve-racking. It makes her movements stiff and awkward. As she starts to stumble toward the water, her foot clipping the edge of the canoe, Lew dashes over to catch her. He keeps her from a hard landing, but almost misses, and they end up a little tangled, with Lew on his knees in the lapping water. Sara jerks back and stands, grateful, but embarrassed. Lew sees a haughty look in her eyes, when he checks to make sure she is okay. He stands, taking off his vest in brisk movements and throws it into the canoe, plainly peeved.

# # #

Nora's body feels so alive, having rowed across a vast expanse of water, overcoming the push of the water, working in sync with her mates. Having their backing enabled her to enter a state of mind she probably could not have achieved had she been out there by herself or with maybe one other person. She could lean into the strength they provided in their group effort, and it freed her mind. She felt a little jumpy at first, but then calm. Looking out over the rolling, almost choppy surface of the water toward the skyline and feeling the constant breezes against her skin was liberating, and she felt she was melding with her surroundings.

Then, Reiko cut in suddenly with a loud, "Look!" And everyone's attention was pulled toward her. A wash of annoyance flooded Nora directed at Reiko, who had yanked her back from the peaceful state she had achieved. "To the left," Reiko shouted again, "a whale!" Her voice was full of delight.

They had no binoculars, but Sister confirmed after a long moment, "Yes, sure enough. See her breach and blow? Quite a ways out, but it is a whale." Excitement flooded Nora, and, for a brief moment, she felt bad about herself for that spike of ill-will.

# # #

Sister encourages them to explore alone and to return to the area in an hour. Later they return near their craft, and show each other what they found, as they settle on the beach to share a meal. Sister has packed guava, berries, nuts, and papaya. Reiko is thrilled to have found some sea glass, and Sara has collected some small pieces of smooth driftwood. Ira brought back some liliko to share, and Sister adds some fruit to his pile.

"Soursop," she says with a smile, pointing to the spiky, green, heart-shaped fruits. Each is a good size, maybe 6 inches long. She cuts them open, and they all taste the delicious sweet-and-sour flesh. Sister explains the medicinal uses of the plant, while they rest on the beach. Sara makes no comment, but her face during this commentary reveals she has opinions. She bites her tongue and holds back from putting in her two cents on the medicinal uses of foods, recalling Lew's acidic response when she shared her knowledge the day before. She puzzles, again, over why he seems to have such a distaste for her and reminds herself to thank him later for preventing her fall from the canoe. She recalls her time at the wishing well this morning when she put in *humility*, and thinks, "Well, here is your opportunity."

They discuss Reiko's sea glass finds: small, smooth, translucent, pebbles of blue and amber—ordinary glass transformed from decades of the ocean's caresses. They remind Reiko of her blue butterfly vision and finding them feels like a good sign.

"Oh, how did I miss that?" Nora says, with a tiny furrow between her brows, as she handles a few of the baubles. Reiko reaches over and takes them from her hand, dropping the pieces back into the little fanny pack she is wearing. She isn't sure why Nora's possessive fingering of her finds is getting to her, but she feels a compulsion to retrieve them. "Sorry," Nora ventures, but Reiko doesn't look at her. Reiko keeps her head down but gives a tight little wordless nod to acknowledge the apology.

"Must be nice," Reiko thinks, gathering her things to get ready to head out. "Having everything a person could want and still looking for more stuff." She'd heard Nora talking about her family over dinner the night before. A nice life. A husband she adores, and three darling little girls. Family nearby who want to help. "Doesn't seem to want for much in that nice little life," she mumbles to herself in a soft whisper, having turned her head away from Nora. She feels bad about the sense of resentment flooding her and knows she should apologize. But not now. She walks over to Sara and admires the driftwood she'd found.

As they gather at the canoe, putting on their vests, Sister speaks in a whisper, so they have to listen closely to hear her, "You are all family this week. All one 'ohana. While you are here, look out for one another, be kind to one another." No one says anything. Sister continues, "'Ohana is family. We are stronger when we work together than when we are trying to work independently. Like we have experienced in the canoe, the paddles must go in at the same time working in unison, or there is no propulsion, and we cannot move ahead, cannot choose our direction."

# # #

The ride back is quick—no shorter than the way out, but their rowing feels easier. They had left the bay and traversed the open ocean a short spell to get to the tiny island. Now they easily move back into the bay. They stop a few times to rest just riding the waves, and Sara relaxes a little, letting her hands drift in the water, cool and yet warm. Everyone feels more relaxed and there is some laughter. Before they know it, they're back where they started in the little cove.

Having disembarked and returned their vests to the canoe, they drop onto the sandy beach to rest. Sister sits among them, and says, "Do you feel the energy in this place? This is where the dolphins come, just as the full moon is beginning and right after. Like now." Sister grins, and continues, "This bay is actually magical. It is in direct alignment with the vortex of Mauna Kea. It is a great place of spirit and healing. A place of nourishment for the soul, a place to heal your heart."

Ira speaks up at that, saying, "That's what it's all about, Sister. Nourishment. We are a piece of the earth; we care for her and she feeds us in turn."

Sister smiles, and nods, saying, "Yes, Uncle, that is true. But there is also another kind of nutrition, which is not on your plate. It is more powerful and important than what you eat. You eat food to fill your stomach, but you have to have relationships and love to feed your soul." Sister's face is full of compassion as she speaks, because she knows how Ira's heart has been broken by his sons.

Sister continues, "Remember when you were a child and you ran and played all day with your friends, never getting hungry. Your parents had to call you in to eat, and you resisted, even though you had not eaten all day. That is because you were nourished from your relationships, and from the love and camaraderie you had with your friends. Your soul was nourished, not necessarily your tummy."

Sister smiles directly at Ira and says, "Our food is our medicine."

'Let food be thy medicine and medicine be thy food.' That is what Imhotep said to Hippocrates, who spread this doctrine to the world."

Lew has been quiet all this time, but now he says, "My father taught me the importance of farming. I never took to it, but I have great respect for farmers. I never thought of food as medicine though."

Sara cannot help herself and pipes up, "There are plants used as food for which there are evidence-based conclusions with indications for certain uses as medication. But I would be hesitant to make such assumptions about any particular plant without seeing conclusions from scientifically based studies. For example—" She sees Lew's eye-rolling expression draped over a heavy sigh, and turns to him a little sharply, "What Lew? Why do my views bother you? No one is stopping you from speaking."

"I just have a little problem with doctors, Sara, and you are one of them. You are all the same. Met quite a few of you in my day. When I finally get an appointment with one of you assholes, you all say the same damn thing. 'Oh, you'll be fine.' Shove a prescription at me and never even look up from your computer. You think you know everything, but you only know anatomy and physiology, oh, and drugs. You don't heal people at all. You have a lot of opinions. Not everyone with stress has the same story or needs the same drugs. I am more than a damn diagnosis. Talk to me sometime and you would find that out." Lew feels his old familiar anger surging through his body, but he remains seated, his body and facial expression giving away more than he knows.

Sara pulls back a little, visibly shaken by Lew's display. Quick, slashing, intense words, and then utter withdrawal. Everyone has fallen silent, and Sara sees Lew's face, his tightened muscles around his neck, as he remains locked in the same seated position. And something clicks for her. He doesn't necessarily dislike her. Well, maybe he does. But he dislikes doctors. A little weight slips off her chest, and her face softens.

Lew keeps his face averted from them all after this exchange. When he finally looks back, he finds Sara sitting apart, gazing out at the ocean, and something about her seems a little different. Odd, she reminds him of his wife with her legs pulled up to her chest, her chin leaning in toward her knees. That bend of her shoulders. The way her hair is blowing around her face. It makes him uneasy. He sees a woman not yet at middle age, a stranger. He really doesn't know her, he has to admit.

But damn if she doesn't give herself away as a know-it-all. Blah, blah, blah. No one came here to listen to all that medical drivel. What good has it done her? No doubt, she has her own stuff going on. Insecure? She is a doctor, so that seems a stretch. But she looks a little fragile at the moment, capable of being hurt. Guess that's just what happens. Hurt people will hurt people.

So much for the *sense of belonging* he put in the well this morning. He'll never find anything like that. He feels an ache in his heart that he associates with home, with Papa and Mama and Isaiah. But he knows it's more than that. It goes deeper. That nugget of pain, lodged deep in his heart, has hardened like a crystal. Why had she given him away? It cuts at him more and more as he gets older.

As a child, he didn't say much about it, because he was afraid of hurting Mama and Papa by talking about her. But recently, with his wife encouraging him to try to find her, he has made some efforts. Had he been orphaned, it would have been painful, but he'd been an innocent baby and *rejected*, right from the start. His own mother had given him away. Now that hurt.

"Sister says nothing but stands and starts to gather loose items into her pack. They all stand and follow her onto the path to head home.

#   #   #

After a dinner of mixed beans, salad, bread, and a fruit salad, they wander outside for their evening gathering. They're all exhausted from a long day of new experiences and the effects of engaging with the open ocean. Darkness is falling fast, and everyone helps get the campfire going before taking their seats on the koa stumps.

After sitting quietly, watching the stars accumulate against a black sky, Sister says, "We're all tired, so we won't gather long tonight. Why don't we hear your experiences today? Reiko?"

"Being on the ocean was amazing. I love to swim, and I've been to the ocean. But I've never done anything like we did today. All day, I carried a sense of anticipation inside my chest, not anxiety, but a joy, not knowing what to expect, yet moving forward anyway. Oh, but seeing that whale! How wonderful."

"Nora?"

Nora replies, "I loved rowing with all of you. I felt like I could focus and achieve something, and still be myself, free in my mind, accepting the support of your strong rowing along with mine. I was thrilled to see the dolphins. And the whale. Thanks for having an eagle eye, Reiko, or we might not have noticed it."

Reiko looks a little embarrassed, but lifts her face toward Nora, "You're welcome. I almost missed it too. But I just felt it there, and I looked over."

"Lew, what about you?" Sister asks.

"Being on the open ocean was the highlight of my day. I love being in open country, running and feeling free. Here I was in the midst of a great open space, but I couldn't act on my own physical need to move through it. At first, it felt restraining, sitting in my place in the canoe. Powerless. I couldn't do anything on my own to make things move. But once we all knew what to do together and rowed out and got the hang of staying in rhythm, well, I felt free again. I felt the power, but I wouldn't have been able to handle that power on my own."

Sister sighs and smiles. "That's the power of 'ohana," she says. "Sara?"

"I learned the same thing as yesterday, I think. I was even more frightened this morning arriving at the canoe and looking out over the bay than I was yesterday getting on my horse. Both times I convinced myself that I would simply refuse to participate in the activity. I would insist I could wait for you guys to get back, and just say no. But riding the horse was really not so hard compared to going out on the ocean. I made myself get on the horse and ended up having an amazing experience. So, I knew that refusing to get into the canoe would be a mistake. I really cannot swim well. But I felt so free out there. And oddly safe also."

"Ira?" Sister asks, "What was most valuable to you today?"

"It felt good to feel a part of a joint activity. Used to be like that on my farm. I was building a legacy and engaging my boys, teaching them. I haven't felt that kind of pulling together in the same direction with other people for a long time. More like pulling away in an unknown direction on my own the last couple of years. It was good to feel my own strength contributing to a team effort toward a solid goal."

Sister responds, "That's good, Uncle. Working together for a common purpose builds heart. And that is what we need to live—community, relationship, heart. Food is nutrition—secondary nutrition—and that is what your life has been about. Food can make us strong, and it can help heal us. Yet, feeding the heart is our primary nutrition. Coming here this week with the parts of your lives that have been undernourished is about learning how to engage *primary nutrition* as a sustaining element in your lives.

"If we fail to nourish our hearts for too long, our hearts fail. A poorly nourished or malnourished heart will not thrive—it hardens, the vessels harden, and inflammation will damage its tissues. That is true in our physical bodies, and it is true in our spirits. *Primary* nutrition addresses the needs of our spirits.

"Sustaining spirit as the nutrition of the soul was practiced thousands of years ago. The principles of the Egyptian goddess Maat were the foundation of ancient Kemet, representing balance, order, law, morality, justice, and harmony. These principles were used both as guides to live by and as means to determine one's eventual resting place in eternity. According to the ancient *Book of Coming Forth by Day*, the heart was valued as the seat of the soul and was not sacrificed in the mummification process. On judgment day, your heart would be placed on the scale of Maat and asked the 42 Negative Confessions, which is similar to the Ten Commandments. If your heart were lighter than the feather of Maat, you were deemed pure and light and could enter the afterlife. If your heart were found to be heavier than the feather, you would be devoured by the jackal god Anubis and taken to the underworld."

Sister looks around for a silent moment at the captivated faces and then asks, "So, any ideas on what would make your heart heavy?" They all appear confused.

Sister continues, "A hardened heart is caused by unforgiveness, guilt, dishonesty, grief, and hatred. These are the things that increase cortisol levels, causing inflammation, elevating blood pressure, enlarging the heart, and causing coronary artery disease."

Sara pipes in, "Oh, now that makes sense. If you look at the heart of a patient with heart disease, the heart is enlarged, so of course it would weigh more. The heart might have plaque with hardened and clogged arteries—"

Uncle interrupts, "which are like stone and would weigh more."

"Exactly," says Sister.

Sara continues, "And a person with heart failure would have a heavy heart because the blood isn't pumping," she says slowly, thinking beyond her words.

Sisters stands and moves toward the open area near the campfire with her arms outstretched. "Let's take from our well." The group joins thumb to pinky and locks in their circle.

Sister starts, "I take out of the well the *pure energy* we experienced, which helped align and sustain us in our journey, as we found the means to support one another." She silently turns her head to Lew.

Lew says, "I take *family connection* out of our well. Families work together, but they don't always get along. Sorry, Sara."

Sara is a little stunned. Now that was unexpected. In a quiet voice, she says, "Thank you, Lew." She realizes after a moment that she is next for the well. "I take out *kindness.*" Taking a deep quiet breath, she adds, "Lew, I don't believe I thanked you for catching me today. So, thank you." She hesitates, but then adds, "It made me feel . . . cared for." She doesn't look at Lew closely, but glances his way with a fleeting smile.

Ira is next and says, "I take out *understanding and forgiveness.* I am getting there, I think. I have to find a way to forgive my sons, and I saw today that I can start by appreciating the gift of forgiveness already given to me by my daughter."

"Nora?"

"I take out *self-esteem.* This morning I put in *neglect,* which is what I have been doing to myself. Handling myself on the open ocean was mind-opening and reminds me what I am capable of—a lot more than I have let myself believe these past few years."

Reiko speaks, once she is sure Nora is done. "I take out *patience with myself.* And that also means patience with others. I have been trying to figure out who I am exactly, and what I want for my life. When I put in my *identity crisis,* that was an understatement. I think I can be a little envious at times. Other people seem to have it all figured out, and I sure don't." She clears her throat lightly, and adds, "I know I also have an apology to make. I hate rudeness. And Nora, I was rude to you today. I am so sorry. I hope you will forgive me."

"Of course, honey," Nora says softly. Reiko doesn't know of Nora's annoyance with her on the boat, and she doesn't tell her. No point. She hadn't known why Reiko's outburst had gotten to her so intensely. "Just like home," she thinks, remembering Kayla's sudden outbursts. Her little girl has a piercing shout and great timing. Nora sighs and sends a good feeling Reiko's way to balance it out.

Sister releases their circle, and makes the gesture indicating stones dropping from a bowl, and they say together, "huli huli."

"I think that is a good takeaway to ponder as we end our day. Let's be patient with ourselves, and with one another, kind to ourselves, and one another. We all deserve kindness. It is our primary food."

Above all else, guard your heart, for everything you do flows from it.

—Proverbs 4:23 NIV

Nutrition Recap

A merry heart does good, like medicine,
But a broken spirit dries the bones.

—Proverbs 17:22 NKJV

Uncle Ira—Broken heart of unforgivingess and grief.

Sister's Solution—Primary nutrition and secondary nutrition. Ira began to understand how to nourish his soul with happiness, relationships, and love, and learns to fuel his body with the most natural source of organic herbs, fruits, and vegetables from Mother Earth.

Nutrition—Promotes heart health, improves mental clarity, and decreases chronic illness. Diet quality affects mental health brain plasticity. Diet during early life is linked to mental health outcomes in children. Manipulation of the diet directly affects cardiovascular health and heart disease.

Chapter Four

Mindfulness/Meditation

In the attitude of silence the soul finds the path in a clearer light, and what is elusive and deceptive resolves itself into crystal clearness. Our life is a long and arduous quest after Truth.

—Mahatma Gandhi

Nora

Nora feels the depth of her breath as her diaphragm opens to accept the fresh island air. She has been hoping for a day like this, focused on meditation and mindfulness. She didn't know that when she came here. Now, it seems to be the reason she has come to this place. Once she knows what she wants, she goes for it. Or at least she used to. At the moment, she is feeling hopeful. She is lying on the soft blanket Sister has laid out for her on a bed of ti leaves in the garden, doing her best to let her body relax and sink into the soft ground.

Her mind fills with thoughts, and she tries to release them, but the thoughts seem to be winning for the moment. She thinks of the lunch they have just eaten. The food Sister serves them is amazing, and that in itself should make her healthier for having come here. She will definitely focus on putting more fresh fruit and vegetables into her family's meals when she returns. And the air here is invigorating. So many hikes and outdoor activities. Why hasn't she done things like that with her crew? Okay, so Grant is never around to take part. But she owes it to the girls to get them into nature.

Back to the breath. Back to the breath. Nora catches herself and lets the thoughts drift away again, drawing in her focus to the breath. Before long, her mind is back to early morning, when they all gathered for their morning circle. Sister had announced their plans for the day, which would start with a hike closer to Mauna Kea right after breakfast. Having the first day's hike in mind and how she had been drawn into a blissful state of mindfulness, Nora felt a sensation ripple through her center—joy—at the thought of another hike like that.

Sister explained how Mauna Kea, though inactive, is a spiritual mountain and that they would be able to feel the positive energy. This is what Nora is after—that connection. She wonders whether there are such places like this near her home, sacred places filled with energy. She'll be sure to ask Sister what she might know about that.

The hike was a little hard for her and some of the others, though not Lew or Reiko. The altitude is so high, the air thin. She took her time on the hike. She was determined to let go and feel the energy, focus on her breath, and be aware of every moment in its fullest. Her pace helped with her breathing as she walked. Oh, right. Breathing. She again pulls her awareness back to the moment and into her breath, riding its movement through her nostrils, throat, chest, and belly, releasing her diaphragm to let it fill.

Sister is speaking again. "Witness your thoughts, let them pass before you."

Nora witnesses her thoughts and releases them. Coming back to her breath, she recalls what Sister told them earlier about breathing.

> In ancient Hawaii, the natives knew the breath was key to good health. It possesses mana, which is spiritual power. The kūpuna, or elders, passed down wisdom by sharing *ha*, which is breath. People greeted by pressing foreheads together and inhaling, as breath was sacred, welcoming a person into their space.
>
> The word *haole* means without breath. It's a derogatory term used even now. **"Ha,"** breath; **"Wai,"** water; and **"I,"** supreme combined as "Hawaii" came to mean "you are the supreme life force, the breath of life." You can connect with the supreme life force that rides on the breath, wherever you are, at any time. If you are upset, breathe. If you are depressed, breathe. The breath will calm and enlighten you. The breath will sustain your health. It is the breath that is life. Honor, respect, value, and trust your breath.

Nora's attention is pulled back to the present by Sister's soft soothing voice.

> "Let's take a few minutes to relax your body and mind. Breathe deeply through your lungs down into your toes. Relax your feet; relax your ankles; relax your calves, your knees, your thighs, your pelvis, and your stomach. Breathe deeply. Relax your eyes; relax your eyebrows, eyelids, eyelashes; relax every part of you, your mind, and your heart. Relax your neck, your ears; relax your body. Relax your lungs; relax your mind, breathe gently as you relax your soul. Thank your body for being here today. Thank your heart for letting go and learning.

"We'll begin with a few slow, deep breaths. Inhale deeply and count to seven, hold the breath for seven counts, then exhale to the count of seven. Do this initially five times to prepare the heart and mind. Each time you breathe in, breathe all the way down into your toes. Breathe in slowly through your nose, and feel your abdomen and lungs expand with air. After drawing in a long, deep breath, allow your breath to flow back out through your mouth. Just let go of each breath, and with it release any tension or stress you might have been holding on to.

"Try this now. Slowly draw in a deep breath. Don't rush to breathe in. Just gradually fill your lungs and abdomen with air, and when they are full, hold it, and then release that breath completely. Pause. You are beginning to feel yourself relaxing. Your breath will dissolve tension just as easily as warm water melts ice.

"Breathe in once again. Feel your body fill with air; hold it—1, 2, 3, 4, 5, 6, 7—and when you are ready, release the breath. Let it flood out naturally. Breathe all the way out until your lungs are empty. Pause. Let's draw in a final breath. Nice and deep.

"Hold it—1, 2, 3, 4, 5, 6, 7. Feel yourself relaxing as you gradually release the breath.

"Now let your breathing return to a normal rhythm, as we begin to scan over your entire body, looking for areas of tension to release. As I mention each body part, I invite you to bring your awareness to it and relax it as deeply as you can. You don't need to concentrate intensely on this task, just feel or imagine a sensation of relaxation and relief moving through each part of your body.

"It's quite common for people to store a lot of tension in their jaw muscles, so let's begin there. Pay attention to your jaw for a moment. There are a number of strong muscles in that area. Just mentally connect with this part of your body and relax it. Allow your jaw muscles to loosen and let go.

"Now let your attention wander to the muscles in your face. Allow your eye muscles to release, and let your cheeks and forehead relax. Let this peaceful feeling flow slowly down your neck. Feel it sooth your throat and dissolve any tension, as it slowly glides down to your shoulders.

"Let your shoulders go. Give them a moment of your attention, and just mentally repeat the word *relax* as you let them soften. Let go and release all tension. Now bring your awareness to your arms. Feel and imagine them becoming loose and limp. They are relaxed and at peace, all the way from your shoulders, through your wrists, to the tips of your fingers.

"Now focus on the muscles in your back. All those muscles surrounding your spine, just let those muscles, relax and let go. Now, bring your awareness to your chest and all the muscles that surround your ribcage. As you breathe in and out, send a mental note to this area of your body, relax.

"As you breathe in and out, feel your stomach gently rise and fall. Let your stomach soften and relax with each breath. Feel it releasing tension, as each moment passes. You can feel yourself slowly slipping into a state of deep relaxation. Now, bring your attention to your thighs. Imagine all those strong supporting muscles beginning to relax and unwind.

Sister's guided meditation continues for about an hour; she allows them to rest for another fifteen minutes before starting to speak again to let them know the agenda for the rest of the day until dinner. Everyone remains slack, splayed on the blankets around the center of the garden.

Then Sister speaks again.

"These past few days, we have explored Mother Nature, the earth, the water, and the wind—through your body and your mind. We have yet to explore the deeper more sacred universe—that which resides in your heart and soul. You will journey deeper into your heart spirit today. Silence will deepen your understanding on this plane and allow you to peer deep within yourself. This is a rewarding, new, open journey with an opportunity to experience who you are, to touch and experience your inward self. Embrace who you can become; cultivate your mind, your ideas; experience yourself in the now, out to the place where you belong.

"Silence will help deepen your understanding of quietness. It will help you achieve some inner peace of your own! We will begin to channel our energy inwardly. This is how all healing begins, from the inside out. That energy we usually direct outward will be focused inward on our hearts. It allows for gentle, peaceful recovery and restoration from our past two days. You will learn it here today, but this you will keep for a lifetime. You can retreat to it when your body calls for rest and renewal. Silence will allow you to go deeper, to the thoughts and feelings that are of utmost concern, which you are choosing to ignore. It will allow you to focus without outside influences, supporting true joy, peace, and happiness. Your thoughts will be quieted, and, eventually, your joyful nature will appear.

"It might take until sunset to quiet your thoughts, to slow the chatter of the noisy thoughts that enter your awareness. Notice them, but allow them to slip away. More thoughts will come like a fussing baby wanting attention. Let them come, notice them, but focus on your breath. As you focus on your breath, you will relax into the quietness. You are creating heightened awareness of your inner and outer world. "You might become frustrated as the random thoughts continue to come into your mind, begging for attention. Breathe, just breathe. Thoughts swing from branch to branch, like monkeys playing in the jungles of your mind. Observe, but don't follow them. These thoughts become less frequent as you continue not to notice them, just let them pass. Don't follow them down that path. Focus on and follow only your breath. Be still, and be aware.

"As with any journey, there are temptations, there are unsafe places. I am giving you a roadmap, a way to get there safely. Just as I pointed the way, on the first day, to the banyan tree, this is the way of the breath. Be patient with yourself, be loving and kind to yourself. This is a journey like no other. The treasures you find will provide riches for a lifetime. Both spirit and soul will be enriched.

"The remainder of the day will be in silent meditation. As you walk, you will notice your breath. There will be no talking or eye contact. I will blow the conch shell for your meal time. We will also eat silently. I will give you further instructions at mealtime on how this will unfold. I am so excited for each of you on your journey today. It will be the beginning of the new you. Remember to walk slowly and breathe. Walk barefoot to allow the energy of the earth to permeate your body.

Sister smiles as she waves. "We begin our day of silence."

Nora is spread out on the ground relaxed, such as she has not felt in years. The last thing she feels inclined to do is move her body from that spot. Nora takes in a long, slow, deep breath, and follows it in and out, in and out, aware of the playful breeze fluttering over her body, her bare arms. The afternoon sun is quite warm; a light scent of flowers is drifting on the wafts of air, and she also tunes into their fragrance, inhaling deeply. She feels feathery and loose, as if she could levitate in air, and it makes her think of the green sea turtle she saw yesterday that stayed with their canoe for a time on the way back from Flat Rock Island. That turtle floating and gliding in the water reminds Nora of how the air around her is making her spirits feel buoyant, light and yet supported.

Honu, Sister had called the turtle, descendant of ancient creatures that guided the Polynesians years ago to the Hawaiian Islands. Swimming great distances migrating through the tropical waters, the honu is the only indigenous reptile found in Hawaii. The honu is a symbol of wisdom and good luck and considered to be a guardian spirit, an *'aumākua*—a family guardian, a personal connection to the ancestors, embodied in the form of an animal.

"So many animals have come and gone over time, and humans are a flash in time compared to the long survival of the honu," Sister had said.

Everything in Hawaii seems to be about spirit and connecting with nature to touch that spirit, Nora thinks. Sister emphasized the need to respect these wonderful creatures. The appearance of a sea turtle might be a call to swim alongside her, but not to touch, as the honu needs to feel secure, and any closer contact would be too stressful.

At this moment, all Nora wants to do is let go of stress, and she envisions herself swimming gracefully through the ocean currents they had rowed over yesterday, with the honu nearby guiding her in a good direction, toward a more nourishing, sustaining sense of family. All of a sudden, Nora hears a wheezy sound, and, sucking in a hard draft of air, she realizes she has slipped into sleep. She laughs to herself, yet holds back from making any noise, remembering she is in silence for the rest of the day. She thinks, *Wow. This is really wonderful. This is incredible. I feel so free. I feel so light. So relaxed. Why haven't I done this before?*

Nora refocuses on her breath. She is now awake, but incredibly peaceful. Her muscles have loosened, and her whole body feels liquid, as if she has melted into the soft ground. Again, a heady floral aroma arouses her sense of smell, and she envisions the abundance of flowers she'd seen in Sister's garden. Nora wonders which of the many varieties is the one that keeps seeking her out. She recalls the hike that morning and all the luscious flowers they had passed, which she had stopped to smell closely a number of times, pressing her face against the soft, velvety petals. She found herself lagging behind the others, with only Sara bringing up the rear. Sara was having trouble with the thin air, as she had informed everyone a number of times. She'd seemed a bit embarrassed about it, yet was often compelled to point it out.

Eventually Nora and Sara caught up with the others. They had stopped to gather at a strange site just off the trail. The site consists of several large, upright stones—an ancient shrine—as Sister explained. She told them these are called heiau, and while they are all over Hawaii, there are many around Mauna Kea. These are sacred sites of great spiritual energy and should be treated with respect. Sister suggested they all remain still and find their center, opening themselves to the feelings and sensations that might be available to them in this place.

Nora felt the energy. A sense of deep peace and happiness, basic and centered, filled her and then remained, even as they continued their hike. The air felt fresher and cleaner, and she heard Ira breathing calmly and deeply. Even Lew seemed less jumpy and not as ready to rush on with hiking as usual. Having opened herself during the entire hike up to that point, she felt like a sponge absorbing the powerful sensations, and was surprisingly humbled by the experience.

The morning hike had lasted only an hour before the group started back to Sister's place. Sister did not think it wise to venture to a higher altitude. They all stayed quiet on the way back, and later, over lunch, Sister explained more about the heiau and its significance.

"Many of them were created for the use of ancient royalty and priests, and some of them are quite large with different forms. There are many smaller heiau, such as the one we visited, which were built by families, though all were shrines and considered sacred. The kūpuna would go there for blessing, and modern Hawaiians still show these sites reverence as an important element in Hawaiian culture."

Nora had felt strengthened by the visit and all the way back to Sister's. She was pleased when Sister announced at lunch they would have a breathing exercise and meditation in the afternoon.

The sweet, floral fragrance is flitting about her face like a butterfly, and Nora feels herself drawn to find it. She stretches languorously and then rolls to her side to sit up. She is in the middle of the garden where they'd gathered the first morning, surrounded by foliage, flowers, bees, and birds. The sky is glorious with masses of puffy, white clouds flowing against a backdrop of brilliant blue—an ideal image as if someone had painted it that way.

She remains seated for some time, looking around her at the beauty of the plants and focusing on her breath. She notices the sensations she is feeling from the air currents, the sun's warmth, and the peaceful feelings inside her body. When she stands, she reminds herself to stay with her breath and makes a point of moving slowly to take it all in.

Nora feels drawn to a large, flowering shrub filled with blossoms, a deep rose color. Another bush nearby has the same kind of flowers, only the blossoms are white with long red stems. She's seen these flowers before. Coming in at the airport, she saw a number of women wearing a single flower behind one ear. Then she notices a plant bearing delicate white petals with a filter of soft pink over the petals at the center, and she rests her face against several of the flowers. The aroma is alluring, intoxicating. This is the scent that has been playing with her all this time, and she stays with it, continuing to breath in its essence.

Sister comes up behind her, humming softly to herself, and Nora turns to her. Sister rests her long hand against her upper shoulder, and reaches over to pluck one of the flowers, deftly placing it behind Nora's left ear. Sister is not taking part in the silence but has said little since they started the day. She speaks now in a low voice, almost a whisper. "I see you're drawn to the hibiscus, Nora. A cherished flower here in Hawaii. It blooms daily, but the blossoms last only a day or two. Feel free to take a blossom or two each day to wear, if you like, the rest of your time with me. And I'll give you some tea made of hibiscus this evening. It has medicinal effects and can have a calming influence on the body." Sister smiles and leaves Nora there to enjoy the flowers, which she does, wandering from plant to plant.

Nora continues wandering in the garden, still drawing attention to her breathing as she goes. She finds her thoughts have their own trajectory, despite her intentions to clear her mind. Witness the thoughts, she thinks. *Witness and release.* And this makes her realize that even thinking these instructions is filling her mind with thoughts.

As she walks, her mind drifts back to arrival day, when she walked up the hill to Sister's place. She was hungry to arrive but didn't quite know why. She had navigated the travel process and slept on the plane—so tired, so angry. It was best to fall asleep rather than focus on how angry she was at Grant. She could have had a career that outmatched his by a mile. She was on track to do so, when she got pregnant, shortly after they'd married. They decided she should stay home awhile, and then, it was never the right time to go back to work. Grant wanted more kids, and it made sense to have their children close in age.

Nora ended up putting all the energy she had for her work into their kids, even homeschooling them to give them every academic advantage. Her life had turned into a swirl of housework, classes, dirty diapers, shopping, sewing Halloween costumes, getting the girls out to social outings and sports, and then supporting Grant's business advancement. He was always kicking ideas past her for her input, and she'd been glad to participate. But she knows darn well, he doesn't give her a shred of credit when he makes use of her ideas.

Then a couple of weeks ago, she'd about had it when she got that call on her cell phone about 3:30, while sitting in the stands at Kayla's soccer practice. Grant wanted her to prepare a dinner by 6:00, so he could bring his boss and a couple of coworkers home to finish up business and seal a deal, trying to impress them. Hardly the first time he had done that to her. She knows he's under pressure too. But somehow all the pressures from his overload, and her own, seem to fall on her to absorb. She is the one who is expected to tie up the loose ends all the time. He barely even notices what he has come to expect from her automatically. No thanks given.

Nora knows Grant is a good man, and he is working hard and trying to live up to his obligations. His long hours and numerous business trips must be hard on him. But when it comes to making a choice between an important home activity and a need of his business, he always chooses business.

Here in this garden, with her mind tuned into a more serene state, she wonders for a moment how she would have handled such choices had she been the one to remain their breadwinner. She always assumed she would have made better, more balanced choices. An urge to reassure herself that, of course, she would have put her family first pushes up in her mind. But she releases that thought and recalls what she was like in college and during her time in the business world. Career was first. No question. She sighs, and then recalls, "Oh yeah, breathe. Breathe."

Nora wanders back to the blanket in the grassy center of the garden where she started and sits on it. Lying back to sink into the ground once again, soon she is back in the taxi the day of her arrival, when, unexpectedly, the driver left her at the bottom of the hill. The man told her he couldn't go any farther on private property, and she got out to walk. She was glad she'd kept her packing light and managed to walk up the winding road, with a bag slung over her back and one in hand.

It was hot, but the sky was so beautiful. And in the distance, she had an amazing view of Mauna Kea. She'd started to cry a little as she walked, recalling Park City in Utah, where she used to go for holiday breaks. And Alta and Snowbird—she used to fly down the powdery trails, a solid skier. Haven't done that in a while, she thinks. That was her life BC—before children. She feels a little guilty, but she knows she loves her kids. She just also needs something for herself.

Recalling now how drawn she was to Mauna Kea right from first sight, she wonders if she sensed its spirit even then. She believes the mountain called to her right then and there, though she didn't think of it that way at the time. Nora feels blessed to have found this place.

She'd known nothing about it, but in the short space of time from when she'd broken down—hopelessly overwhelmed and weeping to her mother-in-law, Pauly—to the time she was boarding a plane to Hawaii, it seemed as if it was meant to be. Pauly had received an email, out of the blue just days before, that included information about a Hawaiian Island getaway, a healing retreat.

"Go on, sweetie," Pauly had implored her. "Go to this place for a week. I really feel it will help you. I love taking care of the girls. I'll keep them busy. We'll have a great time. Please go." Grant was already out-of-town on the second phase of his business trip that was supposed to have included the family. It didn't take any more to convince her. Looking back, she realizes she had sensed something— she did know there would be something for her here.

# # #

They have gathered for dinner, around the large table in Sister's dining room, before the food is placed. They remain in silence and attentive to their breaths, though they had a light lunch and some stomachs are rumbling. The aromas of food are wafting, and the freshly baked bread is particularly enticing.

"So, we will continue our silence as we share our dinner," Sister says in a low voice. She continues to speak.

> "How we eat is just as important as what we eat. Even the healthiest food can harm the body if we do not ingest, chew, and digest properly. Eating in silence will continue to allow the inner voice to guide you. That inner voice remembers the food of our ancestors and will remind you of the healthy choices and food types that have served us for millennia. Your heart

and your intuition have memory embedded in your DNA to support, nourish, and help you thrive to fulfill the purpose of your existence on this plane. Gratitude before you begin and after you eat is the key to a happy life.

"I will place a raisin in your hand, and I want each of you to eat it when I ask you to do so. I want you to chew it thirty times, savoring the flavor, texture, and taste. Experience the raisin, its hard texture. Saliva moistens to release flavor, chewing breaks it down, and the hard part is now soft. Understand the different phases.

"Eating in silence helps us to relearn listening to our inner voice, which knows exactly what we need and when. We come back to ourselves and our individual needs and have the possibility to explore our individual relationship with food and the process of eating. Be grateful for that which nourishes you. Be aware of the person who planted, the person who watered, and the person who picked this raisin. The universe that allowed it to grow, and the person who allowed you to have it.

"Know where your food comes from and understand the health it will give you. There is great happiness, which we sometimes forget in our rush to eat. When we take time to sit and enjoy every morsel of our food, we know we are fortunate to be nourished and embraced by the universe. Put your utensil down after each bite. Be mindful to eat in moderation. Smile in gratitude, supporting one another with nourishing thoughts to feed us on the path of love and understanding."

Sister asks Lew and Reiko to help her put the serving platters and bowls on the table. The meal is quiet, and mostly they avoid communicating with one another, except Lew, who finds it amusing for some reason.

Nora is a little annoyed when he makes some odd faces or points at his plate after taking a bite and putting down his fork. He even kisses his fingertips, as if praising the taste of the food, and Reiko seems to crack up a little, but keeps from laughing out loud. Sara seems about as annoyed at him as Nora is feeling, but she sees Ira does not even notice. He is taking Sister's instructions seriously to give his full attention to the eating process and the food.

Nora really doesn't "get" Lew and generally doesn't care. She is here for her own reasons, and if she makes a friend or two, that is fine. But she came here to get in touch with herself, her true self, and she plans to stay focused on that. She is in no position to judge him and lets it slide. But, for some reason, Reiko's participation in the distraction aggravates her, and then she gets mad at herself for letting Reiko get to her. Reiko didn't do all that much, yet Nora feels herself responding negatively. She turns away, determined to just pay attention to her own meal and keep everyone on the periphery for now.

The meal expands to more than double the usual time. Over the past two days, they would sit around the table and chat after they were done eating. Tonight, they remain seated in silence and get up when the last napkin is dropped to a plate. Sister asks them to remain in silence until they gather for their evening circle, and also asks for a couple of volunteers to assist with kitchen clean-up. Uncle Ira and Reiko both raise a hand and clear the table.

# # #

"Sara, tell us about your day," Sister says softly, inviting an end to the hours of silence. Darkness has not fully fallen. They'd made a campfire in silent cooperation, and its vigorous crackling was the only sound until Sister spoke.

Sara seems a little surprised to be called first and clears her throat. "Well, that was strange. I usually have a lot to say, but after staying quiet for so long, I feel like I have less to say. It was mostly calming. I certainly noticed a lot more—small things, details I don't normally bother with. Here's something: I am not really a dog or cat person, no pets at home. But as I was sitting on the edge of the garden for several hours, your cat came out of nowhere and jumped in my lap. Surprised all heck out of me. But I managed to stay quiet. Then she just turned in a circle and kneaded my thighs for a while before settling down for a nap. It was nice."

Sister said, "Kiwi is picky about whom she chooses to spend her time with. She must have sensed something from you that made her feel your lap was a good choice." Sister smiles, and adds, "Okay, now tell us something about the day that didn't go well."

Sara makes a slight face, then says, "Well, getting up the mountain this morning was difficult. I really think it is the thin air, as you've pointed out, Sister. I'm not in great shape, but that was really hard. I enjoyed the shrine, ah, the heiau, but I can't say I sensed anything unusual there. It was interesting. And I had a hard time sitting still for so long. I know I could have walked or run," she says, glancing at Lew, "but mostly I found walking distracting, so I sat. And I did pay attention to my breath. Lots of thoughts and distractions. I feel relaxed now, I do. But," she gives her head a little, skeptical shake, "I don't really see myself doing that in my regular life."

Sister nods and says, "Thanks for sharing, Sara."

Sara adds, "I just want to say though, and I don't mean to be critical, but whether I agree or not with any particular exercise, I think we should try to stick with it. I did feel myself getting rather distracted by you at dinner, Lew. I know you meant it as fun. Just saying, though."

If Lew had a reaction, Sara didn't notice, as she didn't turn her head toward him, and he didn't say anything.

"Okay," Sister says, "Ira?"

"Great day, Sister. I enjoyed the mix of exercising my body and relaxing it. I loved visiting the heiau. I've been to sites like that before, but this was different. My mindset was different. And I haven't enjoyed a meal like that in a long time. Thank you. I didn't really have anything that was negative, although it was a little hard hiking at that altitude. Oh, right, and I did have thoughts intruding during my silence; some made me a little sad. But I worked with it."

"Reiko?" Sister says.

"I had a wonderful day, Sister. I felt the energy at the mountain and was buoyed by it. I love the walking. Such a beautiful place to be. Butterflies everywhere. I felt myself floating at times. I loved the period of silence. It feels natural to me, and I spent a lot of the day walking around. When I was young, my home was near my grandparents, who live this way.

Sister says, "Okay, anything that was hard for you?"

Reiko thinks a moment and says, "Well, I thought about my grandparents. They came up in my mind a number of times. They live peaceful and humble, in Japanese tradition. I remember the quiet love they showed me. I remembered how much I miss them. I've tried so hard to please them and my parents. I am trying to find my own way in the world, but I still need them and the rest of my family. It made me a little anxious that I could lose my family."

Sister nods, and turns her head to Lew, "Lew? What stands out for you?"

Lew shifts his position a little and leans forward, "Not my thing, I guess. The silence and the breathing stuff. I stuck with it when I could, and I was afraid you'd ask us to sit there all day. So, when you told me I could run while I did it, as long as I focused on my breath, well, that was okay. I ran a good part of the day, just a nice steady pace, with lots of rest stops. I did keep coming back to the breath, but my mind was not really calm. No, I wouldn't say that. So, the good part—running. The heiau was cool too. The bad, well, not being able to talk when I want to just say something. And then, people who get bent out of shape when everything doesn't fit into the neat little categories they have in their own minds. *Just saying.*"

"Nora," Sister says, "how about you?"

"I had a really good day, Sister. I think this breathing thing, this energy thing, is important to me. It might be the reason I'm here. I can't say I did it all that well. My brain is active, and when I relax my body, it seems my mind really kicks into high gear sometimes. But I worked with that, and when I became aware of it, I drew my focus back to my breath. I loved the heiau. I want to learn more about them. I loved the energy there. I felt peaceful and strong, and it stayed with me. I wonder about the energy sites, Sister. Are they on the mainland also, or just here?"

"They are found in many places around the world, Nora. We can talk about that later, if you like. So, anything negative?"

Nora paused, "Well, I thought a lot about my life back home, the problems that drove me here. That is what would come up when my mind went off on its own, away from my attention to my breathing. So that would agitate me a little. When I go home, I still will have to deal with all that stuff, and I haven't yet figured out how to make changes.

And without meaning to be difficult, I would second what Sara said about distractions."

The group falls quiet. After a moment, Sara says, "Sister, I am really trying to understand, and I can see where the experiences I am having here are helpful. Certainly, the exercise and trying new things, like horseback riding and canoeing on the ocean. Never would I have pictured myself doing that! I feel it has opened me up, and I have to say I feel a lot more relaxed than when I left Knoxville. But you haven't backed up some of your claims about medicinal uses of plants or breathing exercises, which are really just a form of meditation. So, I have a hard time just accepting those things at face value."

No one says anything, although all of them, except Lew, feel a little embarrassed by her comments. Lew is not embarrassed but angry again and feeling vindicated that his initial assessment of Dr. Sara wasn't off the mark in his view. But he keeps his mouth shut out of respect for Sister.

Sister speaks up. "Well, Sara, I can understand that. You have studied medicine and science for a long time and your worldview has been shaped by that. There is truth in what you say. The knowledge I am making available to all of you is based in ancient wisdom that is reinforced in each generation and can be used to help us live full and happy lives. Much of it has passed down by oral tradition, but the results are consistent.

"On the other hand, there are studies that have been done, which do support many aspects of what I have to teach. The science behind the breathing exercise is that slow, deep breathing stimulates the vagus nerve, which courses along the diaphragm. This stimulates the parasympathetic system to relax. So be patient, we still have time together this week. I hope you will find something that will help you improve your life when you return home."

Sara says, "Oh, of course, Sister. I am open to learning from you. I have gotten a lot out of my time here so far, as I said."

"Nora, tell us about your discovery of the hibiscus."

"I just felt drawn to it. I wasn't aware of it so much, though once I noticed it, I realized they are all over the place. I saw women wearing them behind their ears before driving out here." She touches the flower in her ear. "I'm wearing it behind my left ear, because I'm married, as Sister explained is the custom. Wearing it behind the right ear is for those available for a new relationship. It was calling me all afternoon, I could smell it out of all the flowers in the garden, as if it was looking for me." Nora laughs a little.

"Lew," Sister says, "I saw you noticing a flower also. It's called the bird of paradise."

"Ah, yeah, strange little flower. Never saw anything like it."

"This flower grows wild in Hawaii and is important to Hawaiian culture. It is about keeping a good outlook on life, a healthy perspective." Smiling, she glances around at the rest of them. "It is incredibly beautiful. Brilliant and multicolored, in the shape of a crane's head. We will come back to our discussion of flowers. Notice which of them you are drawn to in the course of your time here."

Sister stands and holds out her hands for everyone to join her at the well. They lock fingers and stand silently, breathing deeply. "Nora," Sister says after a long moment, "what would you like to take from the well?"

"*Self-appreciation.* This morning I put in *self-denial*, as I never take time to care for myself; mostly I just run, run, run trying to keep up with my family's needs. Having this time away from them is allowing me to see how I've ignored myself. Especially tonight, eating in silence and mindfulness made me realize there are lots of times I never even make it to my seat at the table back home. I'm up and filling plates and tending to a million details. I've been gaining weight and feeling lousy, and it's no wonder why." Nora has a catch in her voice that makes it clear she's feeling emotional. "I came to understand that I haven't loved myself for a long time. I used to. Today, I felt myself again, like I had to come so many miles from home to find myself."

Sister nods, and says, "Yes, it is not one-dimensional, the mind, body, and spirit. You need to love yourself and not judge yourself. Appreciate who you are for yourself, and not just as your family's caretaker. Regardless, you do them more good, have more to offer your loved ones, when you *first* fulfill your own needs and appreciate your own value, as yourself."

Sister turns to Lew. "Lew, how about you?"

"Well, I take out *relaxation*. My brain is always so active, so much going on all the time, I never just sit and relax. I put in *anxiety* because that is the constant backdrop in my life, this feeling that something could go wrong at any moment. And I always seem to have a sense of something being missing, but today, I did move through a lot of that static."

Lew remembers, again, his wife urging him to look for her. Mama had been more than happy to help him and gave him the name she'd recalled—Lucinda Luvenia. He managed to trace her to a phone number, but then the trail went cold. Well, he hadn't pursued it further, really. He wonders why he'd never had the courage to keep trying after that. At the moment, he feels his intentions forming around this need again, and he knows he will keep looking.

Sister turns to Ira and says, "Uncle, what do you take out?"

Ira says softly, "*Peace*. I take out peace. I put in *guilt*, and I think I am coming to understand that forgiveness moves in many directions. I've had trouble forgiving my sons, and I have felt guilty about how I had overlooked my daughter, and so grateful that she has forgiven me. And guilty that I had not been able to connect with my sons to the point that I never saw their actions coming. I blamed myself as much as I blamed them. I am feeling more and more that I won't be able to really forgive the boys until I forgive myself. My wife was a forgiving person; actually, she was slow to blame anyone in the first place for much of anything. I spent a lot of time with memories of her today. I feel peaceful."

Sister nods at Reiko.

"I take out *patience*. Today, in slowing down, I remembered the still place already inside me, and by going inward, I was able to connect with so much around me. At one point, I recall just watching a leaf floating from a branch to the ground, and I became that leaf somehow. I could feel myself floating, and I felt good, as if being a part of nature and all its goodness made me whole and worthy. I am young and single and valuable for who I am, as I am. I am finding a well of patience inside me to just let that unfold."

Sister nods with a smile, and then turns to Sara.

"I take out *understanding*," Sara says softly. "I have not understood a lot in my life, and I know I haven't. But I haven't known how to put my finger on what it is I am missing or how to find it. I just feel like I am locked away inside my head all the time. And that was not so different today. Most of the day, my thoughts churned as usual, and I would bring them back to my breath. But by the time I heard the conch shell for dinner, I was starting to feel my mind easing up. I got a small sense of what I have been missing, an inkling of myself beyond all the chatter inside my brain. And I stayed with it. Even when getting up to walk in to dinner, I walked slowly, and stayed with my breath."

Sister nods and says, "And I take from the well the joy of feeling your energy expand with your own actions today, freely opening yourself to new possibilities of how to be more fully yourselves."

Sister sits back on her stump, and the rest of them follow suit.

"It is difficult to drive while focusing on the rearview mirror. Inevitably, you will crash. Look forward through the window to see that which awaits you. Look at the journey that lies ahead. Take each day as a present and drive in destiny on the road to life. It is wide and expansive. And you can travel faster with your foot off the brake.

"Today was challenging. Today you forced yourself to get in touch with the person you love to avoid—yourself. I am sure there were periods of confusion, frustration, and anger. So, thank you for persisting and succeeding in discovering the new you."

Sister stands and makes the now familiar gesture of turning over a bowl with one hand. "Huli huli," she says softly and turns to leave them, with a gentle wave of her hand.

Talking comes by nature, silence by wisdom.

—A proverb

Mindfulness/Meditation Recap

The best way to capture moments is to pay attention. This is how we cultivate mindfulness.

—Jon Kabat-Zinn

Nora—Lost herself in the midst of motherhood.

Sister's Solution—Self-reflection, work on the breath, meaning of Hawaii, silent meditation.

Mindfulness—Reduces anxiety, reduces implicit age and race bias, might prevent and treat depression, increases body satisfaction, improves cognition, helps the brain stay focused with less distraction. Yoga and meditation practices exert positive influence on addictive behaviors.

Chapter Five

Massage

Many people are alive but don't touch
the miracle of being alive.

—Thích Nhât Hạnh

Sara

"Lomi lomi massage," Sister says to the group gathered around her on the koa stumps for their morning gathering. "It fell out of favor, or actually had to go underground when the Westerners, the Christians, came. They outlawed many ancient traditions because they didn't understand them, labeling them as heathen practices. So traditional Hawaiian massage was forbidden, but it has survived. I am fortunate, indeed, to have had good teachers who passed on this healing practice to me.

"It is a massage of touch, but it also has to do with touching memories. Lomi lomi was traditionally given to adults and children. If a child was sick, the child was given lomi lomi, because the child's body had taken on bad spirits, and the massage would change the energy of the young one to drive away this bad energy. It would be done by hands through massage, but also by chanting and saying a prayer for whatever the hopes and intentions were for the person receiving the massage.

"Massage reaches deep inside us to heal. Every cell in the body has memories; the issues are in the tissues," Sister says with a slight smile. "Old memories, behaviors, and patterns can get locked into our body, and if their energy is negative, they create stumbling blocks in our lives. Lomi lomi releases this energy from our cells, helping to remove the hidden root causes of what might be preventing us from living our lives fully and joyfully. By releasing these fetters, it brings hidden patterns out into the open to be faced; and, ultimately, we are able to grow and move past them."

Lew is visibly uncomfortable once Sister makes it clear she is offering them lomi lomi massage. Uncle Ira turns his face toward the garden entrance and looks like he would just as soon slip into the garden for the rest of the day. Ira says, "Never had a massage, Sister. Well, other than from Dottie, my wife. She rubbed my neck and shoulders sometimes after I pulled a muscle or something like that. I don't think it is something I really want to do."

"Well, Uncle," Sister replies, "I respect that. I would like you to have the experience of lomi lomi, as it is unique. Why don't we just do a hand or foot massage? Would that be okay?"

He doesn't say much, but seems a little embarrassed at the thought, and gives a small noncommittal shrug.

"Tell you what, think it over, and we can discuss it later. I'll start with anyone who wants to volunteer." All three women raise a hand, and Sister says with a nod toward Sara, "Sara, you can go first."

Sara stands and starts to follow Sister into the garden, but then asks her to wait a moment while she retrieves something from her room. Sister lets the others know when to expect their turn. They agree that Nora and then Reiko will follow. Then, after a few minutes, Sara reappears.

Sara trails after Sister, stepping with her usual tentative footfalls, walking barefoot on the thick grass. She is unusually quiet today and hasn't communicated much, other than to raise her hand for the massage. Once again, she had to push past her internal barriers and voices of caution, but by her fourth day here, she has learned better than to turn down the opportunities she is being offered by Sister. Accepting them has turned out to be the right decision, by far. And she wants the massage, as much as she is full of trepidation at the thought of its intimacy. She hasn't been touched by anyone other than Isaac for years, except for her kids, and an occasional hug or pat on the arm by a friend.

They arrive at an alcove enclosed by trees and low shrubs on the outer reaches of the garden, a shady area that Sara has not seen until now. There are a couple of carved wooden chairs off to the side and a small table with a bowl and a large container wrapped in towels. In the center of the space, there is a table, not exactly a massage table, but it is long enough to hold a person. Sister holds out a hand indicating she should lie down on it. "You should loosen or remove your clothes to whatever extent you're comfortable, Sara."

Sara slides out of her blouse and slacks, and it is apparent that she had run into the house to put on her bathing suit under her clothes. She folds her top and slacks neatly in half and lays them in a large basket placed on the grass near the chairs, and then she lies down on her belly. Sister places a large towel over her.

"Now, Sara, I understand you haven't had a massage before, so we're going to start at your head and work our way down. If there are any areas you're not comfortable with, just let me know," Sister says as she places oil in her hands from a bowl nearby.

Sara turns her head slightly to the side and nods. Then, after a moment, she feels Sister's lengthy, strong hands rest gently on her head. She begins massaging her head, giving her scalp a massage, traveling in circular motions with her fingers and palms. Sara has to catch her breath at first. She wasn't sure what to expect, but this feels marvelous. So relaxing, and oddly energizing, probably from the increased blood flow to the area, she concludes. But it is oh, so good.

Sara said nothing when Sister said she understood she had not been massaged before, quietly remembering she had a massage on her honeymoon. It was an odd experience. Her husband got the idea from reading brochures in their hotel room, seeing that the hotel spa offered couple massages as part of the amenities. She resisted, but he talked her into it, and she went along, not wanting to seem too stuffy. He actually liked it, but she had a terrible experience. It was a deep-tissue massage delivered by a masseur who dug into her body with hard, probing pressure, saying it would release tension. She was sore for the next two days. She had vowed—no more massages. And now, here she is getting a massage.

This is not the same thing. She realizes that fairly quickly, to her relief. Sister's pliant fingers move down from her head to her neck and shoulders, and then shift upward again, focusing on the back of her head. Sara has had a lot of migraines over the years. When Sister concentrates on that area for a long time, it feels superb. The light floral scent of the oil on Sister's hands is delightful. She eventually slides down her neck and shoulders and spends a lot of time on the entire cervical region of her back. Then the thoracic and lumbar regions too, working along her entire spine. Sara falls asleep, and Sister continues massaging her legs and feet, then her arms and hands, pulling along each finger and toe.

Sara wakes suddenly as Sister is finishing her feet. She has Sara turn onto her back, and then returns to her head, rubbing her temples, and around her eyes and cheeks. Sara says, "Oh, my gosh. I've never had any massage like this. It's so relaxing, just incredible. I actually did have a massage one time, Sister, but it was not a good experience. Too rough. Nothing like this."

Sister tilts her head toward her and touches Sara's arm. "Just lie her for a while and rest. Take it in. We have a little more to do." Sara nods, grateful to be able to stay put for now. Sister takes a seat near the head of the table and sits quietly.

Sara closes her eyes and remembers she'd fallen asleep; she feels a little embarrassed. But then, an image comes into her mind, and she is back in her dream. She is young, and she is with her grandma. Sara always feels so close to Gran, so much warmth. She encircles Sara with tenderness. Gran has a lot of family. Ten children and lots of grandkids. But Sara always feels like she is Gran's favorite. Sara is looking up at the aunts and uncles around her, when her dad scoops her up, saying, "Sweetie, your granny wants to see you. She said she wants to see her tweetie-pie." Daddy holds her over Gran's bed, saying, "Go on, honey. Lean over and give Granny a hug. Granny needs a hug, baby. That'll make her feel better."

Sara sees Gran's eyes light up with pleasure at seeing her, and Sara just has to get to Gran. She wants to wrap her arms around Gran so badly. Gran will let her lie with her for a while. She is a little sleepy, and oh, to snuggle in with her Gran and rest awhile. Daddy has a tight grip on her, but Sara squirms hard to get free, and she slips from Daddy's grasp, falling into bed with Gran. Right on top of her stomach! Gran lets out an awful yelp, and Sara feels horrible.

"Gran, I'm sorry! I'm sorry!" She starts to cry, even though Gran is the one who's gotten hurt. But Sara can't help crying. She can't stand the thought she's hurt Gran. Gran just smiles at her and shakes her head gently.

"Don't worry, baby. I'm fine. Shhh." Sara's dad picks her up and stands her on the floor. He bends down to comfort her and says, "Gran's okay, baby. It's not your fault." Then, off she goes, hand-in-hand with her older cousin, Karen, who is asked to take her in the other room, where she continues to sniffle over it.

Gran died a few days later, and Sara believed she caused it. Daddy had said she would be able to make her feel better, and just the opposite happened. Gran died of colon cancer. She would have died anyway, whether or not Sara had fallen on her, but Sara believed she hastened her death. The emotional wallop of believing she had caused Gran's death at that tender age had stayed with her. That moment had a certain feeling, and it would just rise up out of nowhere sometimes and haunt her.

She decided as a child to become a doctor. It was tied to losing her Gran, she knew. Sara determined she was going to help people; she didn't want anyone to become sick and suffer. She became devoted to that ideal of healing. She recalls the satisfaction she felt when she took her oath upon becoming a doctor. And it means every bit as much now as then, even if she has lost some enthusiasm for the job itself.

She really wants to heal people to the best of her ability, but she never could bring herself to touch them. She did extremely well in school, bright and promising. She knows a great deal about the art of medicine, but she never touches her patients. She knows people always end up thinking of her as standoffish, aloof. She's had complaints. A number of them. People think she's stone cold, even though she tries to show kindness. But something inside her makes her feel that she would cause them pain or hurt people just by touching them. She never can quite believe a touch from her would even be welcomed by anyone. Though she really does care, passionately. She cares so deeply that she ends up carrying around the pain she imagines her patients are feeling and longs to take that away.

Add to those difficulties the mountains of digital and paper records, forms to complete, and it just wears her down. She is too tired to find the emotional strength to even try to keep up with it all. She would leave the hospital and find another way to use her education, but she can't. Not yet. Not until the school loans are paid down. She sighs heavily.

Sara feels Sister place her hands on her head again and begin softly running her fingers in gentle circles around her temples and forward. "It's all right, Sara. Just let it go. Let it go. You want to heal people. I feel how much you want to heal. You need touch. You need to touch people. You need to let them touch you. You care, but touch is the way to let people know you care, so they can accept your healing energy. You can touch them with your heart. Putting a hand on a shoulder means the world to someone in need of healing."

Sister slides her hands down to Sara's shoulders and continues the massage. Sara can feel tears sliding down both her cheeks and she keeps her eyes closed, as she accepts the healing Sister is directing to her. Demonstrating for Sara what she needs to give her patients. "You need to let go and forgive yourself, heal yourself. And then you can move on and give others your gifts."

Then, Sister whispers, "She moved on, you know. You helped her transition. You helped give her the peace to move on, and then she was free of her pain. It was time. She loved you, and you know her leaving was not because of you. It was her time."

Sara opens her eyes and looks into Sister's with a slightly tender look. Sister smiles and places one long finger up to her own lips and shakes her head softly. "You see, Sara, what is involved with touching. It is the greatest gift a healer can give, and receive. It is a two-way path. It is not about knowledge alone, but the ability to connect. And that is the most direct way human beings connect. It surpasses other communication."

Sara takes a deep breath, and says on the exhale, "But how do you know how to connect?"

Sister raises her shoulders a little and drops them lightly, "I just do."

Sister asks Sara to lay on her stomach again. "I have one more thing to do with the lomi lomi," she says. When Sara turns over, Sister draws smooth flat stones from a clay pot she had wrapped in several towels and places them one at a time along Sara's spine. The intense warmth spreads deeply into Sara's spine and the surrounding tissues, and a sense of sweet relaxation and release spreads through her body. She feels calmed, after having cried for a while thinking of Gran, and about how she had always blamed herself deep inside for her death. She is still wondering how Sister could know any of it. She notices the bowl of essential oils Sister has been using for the massage, and sees a few small white flowers floating in it. It has a lovely fragrance, which filled her senses as she was receiving the massage.

"What are the flowers in the oil, Sister?" Sara asks in a quiet voice.

"Those are pikake, Sara," Sister replies. "They are a form of jasmine. Leis are made of them. They are used to welcome people into your life. Pikake are used in aromatherapy to encourage optimism and rejuvenation, restoring positive energy. These all help to restore your body, mind, and spirit. As I said yesterday, we are not one-dimensional and need to address all parts of our being."

After a while, Sister takes the stones back and returns them to the pot. Sara sits up and gradually puts her clothes on. As they get ready to walk back to the house, Sister holds her hand out to Sara, and Sara hesitates only a second before taking it, and then, stepping forward, she gives Sister a hug. A quick hug. But a hug, nonetheless.

# # #

Nora recalls her best friend, Nancy, who had given her an amazing gift, and how she had not used it. In retrospect, it makes her sad to think she did that to her friend. But even more so, she cannot believe she bypassed the opportunity to have a spa day at that exquisite facility. She didn't realize how much it had cost her friend—$500! She found out months later.

Having just had the most amazing massage of her life and now resting on the thick grass near the hibiscus plants in the garden, she realizes how incredibly relaxing and delightful it would have been for her to accept her friend's gift with good grace and to just enjoy it. She looks back and recalls how she had believed she did not have a minute to spare in her life at that time. And now, she sees the truth of it—she wasn't loving and valuing herself to be worth such a luxury. That was the true root of her decision.

So, she gave it away to another friend, Ellie, a woman she used to work with. And a few weeks later, she got a call from her. "Nora, I don't know why you gave me this gift, but it was the best thing I've ever had in my life. Thank you, dear." Nora had been a little surprised at that, instantly wishing maybe she had kept it. And she couldn't tell Nancy she hadn't had her spa day, so it was a little awkward. Anyway, massage is now one more thing she can take home with her and use to maintain her balance when life feels hectic. She'll invite Nancy and make it up to her. They will have a spa day together.

# # #

Reiko has needed that touch, and it is freeing for her. She knew right away she wanted the massage as soon as Sister started talking about lomi lomi. She has been in such a state of anxiety. Today, Sister's touch while massaging her makes her feel light, liberated in some way. Always these feelings make her think of butterflies now, and she feels the transformation a little at a time, and this is just one thing more contributing to that feeling.

Reiko has had massages, so she understands this is different. She feels cleansed somehow and strengthened. She tries to express these feelings to Sister after the massage, and Sister listens, then replies, "Reiko, it speaks to your soul. That is done by sharing your mind, body, and spirit in this unique touching; it is in the way it is done. It is strengthening, at all those levels. For one who is ill, but also for one who is well and healthy, as you are. You are finding yourself, and there is so much there to find. Remember you are a butterfly. You are a beautiful and thoughtful free spirit. You don't need to be a part of anyone's group. You are the group. You can go anywhere and do anything because you are uniquely you." Sister smiles, and the energy she is sharing with her is palpable.

# # #

Ira is glad to have a day with minimal activities, and now he is back in the garden to enjoy the rest of it. He hung around for the foot massage, and now, all in all, he is glad he did. It was so relaxing, he felt himself nodding off, and it went on for quite a while. His mind kept drifting to Dottie, while Sister was massaging his feet.

Dottie's been on his mind a lot lately. He's missed her so much since she died that he's found it too painful to dwell on memories of her. He would stop himself whenever his mind would drift there. But today, he was with her, and it made him emotional. He didn't start crying, for which he was glad. Letting someone give him a massage didn't feel too manly to him, and tears would have proved it to everyone. So, he just let himself be there, with Dottie, and feel the way he had felt with her back then. It felt so good, and he thinks it is time to remember her again, not as a painful memory, but a cherished one. Yes, it is time. He can do that now.

Ira loves this garden of Sister's. It is something he dreams of having. Being here, seeing it as a reality, somehow is making him believe he could also do this. Sure, the soil here is better than back home, but the Hawaiian soil is wonderful no matter where. It's strange, as much as he loves the idea of this magnificent garden, while he had the farm and was focused on production and care of a few crops, he would never had made the time or space to create such a dream.

He realizes that the loss of his farm, which has been so devastating to him, in a way has opened up some room in his mind to follow his heart. Ira forms his intention right then and there. He will create his own healing garden. There are many things he can do to make it self-sustaining. He knows a lot about the plants, and perhaps Sister will enlighten him further on medicinal uses. There's no reason he couldn't sell some of his healing plants to support it all.

Ira is now walking the garden with more purpose, taking notes from Sister, who has joined him there, as she points out the healing plants and tells him what she knows of them. "Noni," she says. As Ira had pointed out to Lew, Sister confirms it has strong healing properties. He walks over and feels the dark green, shiny leaves. They are deeply veined; Sister comments they are used topically to treat skin problems. And the fruit pulp is used internally for worms, but also for other ailments. He'll have to study up.

She shows him 'olena, turmeric, also for skin sores and rashes, and for nasal passages. But he's heard it burns like hell, so he wouldn't use it that way. Ira keeps walking, and Sister points out kukui, a candlenut tree. He remembers his elders using it as a purgative whenever anyone had constipation. And he remembers talk of using it to relieve babies' pain from teething. Sister smiles and says, "The nuts taste good when roasted too. The root bark of *uhaloa* is for sore throats." She gestures, as they pass the gray-green shrub. "And *awapuhi*, wild ginger, which was brought by the ancient Polynesians and is growing most everywhere, treats stomach ailments and such."

Ira is feeling excited, a renewal of focus such as he has not felt in some years. "My healing garden," he thinks. "Mahalo, Sister."

#   #   #

Lew contemplates the massage. He really did not want a massage from Sister, even though everyone else had received their massages; he's had all morning to consider it. He finally decides that it would be a mistake to not listen to Sister, as she has been right about so many things. He knows the women have gone for full body massages, but that's a bridge too far for him. Even a foot massage seems intrusive, although Uncle Ira seems to have come through it well enough and has now wandered off. Lew's been jogging through fields most of the morning, but he's back in time for his turn. When Sister mentioned a hand massage, well, he figured he could handle that.

He follows Sister back to an alcove hidden in the garden. He hadn't noticed it, and he's an observant guy. He settles in a small chair carved of koa wood, and Sister sits in front of him, taking his hands in hers. She starts rubbing the inside of his palms with the pads of her thumbs, which she's dipped in some essential oil. He feels an overwhelming sense of letting go. It alarms him a little, and he takes a deep breath and tries to pull himself together. But she smiles and keeps moving her thumbs and then the rest of her fingers, enclosing his large hand in hers.

"Take some deep, slow breaths, Lew," Sister says softly. "Relax the way you did yesterday during our breathing and relaxation session." Sister repeats some of the directions she had given yesterday for relaxing the entire body, part by part. And Lew feels himself being pulled in and out of the tides, rolling on her low, warm voice.

His mind focuses on the sensation of his hands securely placed in hers, and it gives him an odd feeling of safety. It makes his throat a little thick at the thought of it. He never feels safe. Sometimes, he is able to make others feel that way. Mostly because of his training and his own strength, which makes it possible for him to offer protection. But no one makes him feel safe. Not even his wife. He feels her concern for him, and her desire to make him feel that way, protected. But he doesn't. He knows providing safety is what he does for others. Yet, Sister's hands feel reassuring, as they press into his flesh. He is embarrassed suddenly, as he feels an urge to cry, and he'll be damned if that is going to happen. But that need rises up in him as an insistence, the way a child feels the urge to cry out at pain or insecurity.

It makes him think of Mama, and how she would hold him when he cried as a young child. And then, he saw another woman, not Mama, not Sister. A woman he has never seen, a shadow. She is looking down at his hands and rubbing them tenderly, and he knows who she is. He cannot speak, but the emotion rises in his chest. All he has felt lacking in his life all this time, the love he has always been convinced he was missing is right in front of him, pulsing with life and energy. And as angry as he has let himself be at her, at her definitive rejection of him, it melts away in this touch. He has been afraid to find her, because she rejected him. But there is no rejection here. Just tenderness. If more rejection is a possibility, well then, this is also a possibility. Tenderness.

Sister notices Lew's energy change. Lew clears his throat to speak, but his words get stuck in his throat. He looks at Sister, and, as their eyes lock, he feels naked and vulnerable. He quickly closes his eyes, as Sister begins to speak softly.

"You are a loving, kind, gentle soul, Lew. You are a great father and a good husband." Sister continues to affirm him. "You are still engaged in daily conflict from which you are trying to flee. Lew, live in the moment. Your past has haunted you long enough. You can't change the past. Focus on your breath. Being a soldier was a part of who you were; it was your training and the mission. You did what a soldier is asked to do. You defended your country, and your service has given us all the liberties and freedom we enjoy today. Live in the moment and don't allow your thoughts to run rampant. I know you are misunderstood and angry about the way the system works. You don't take it out on society or your family; you take it out on yourself."

Lew's mind drifts to a time at the VA clinic when he'd had an argument with the nurse who rudely questioned him during his disability rating interview. *What does a damn wounded vet look like? he'd thought, an ole man in a wheelchair with an American flag in his hat?* Then he had blurted out, "Bitch, I told you, I can't sleep, and I can't keep a damn job. Maybe you need to get a fucking new one, 'cause you sure as hell ain't doing this job well!" He stormed out without his meds. No worries, he could easily get a dime bag and what he needed from a friend.

Sister's voice brings him back. "Lew, you have struggled for some time. The bravery you showed on the battlefield pales in comparison to the courage you have shown daily in trying to get your life back. Forgive yourself, Lew. Forgive your past, and what you couldn't do, and what you couldn't control. Begin today to live in your present, appreciating the journey you are on. Relish the fun and laughter of your boy, Solomon, and the compassion and love of your wife. Prepare for your future as a good father, a courageous man and devoted husband. Change the lens with which you are viewing the world.

"You are eating fresh fruits and vegetables, feeding your body here. You are moving in Mother Nature and exercising purposefully. Trust your heart, not your mind. Focus on living in the present moment because really that is all you have—your breath."

Somehow able to touch the child-spirit in this man, Sister gently finishes the massage and quietly leaves Lew to his thoughts and his tears.

# # #

They all gather again outside for their evening circle, well before sunset. No one has spoken much today. Everyone is relaxed and easygoing having had their massages. Reiko and Nora also spent a good part of their day focused on remaining quiet and engaging in breathing exercises. Uncle Ira has spent the day walking the gardens and examining the plant life. Lew seems relaxed, even subdued. Sara has spent some time in her room writing, and then several hours out in the garden focusing on her breathing.

Sister has been reminding them off and on all day to stay hydrated to continue removing toxins. She has talked about the importance of being aware of their surroundings and how their bodies are feeling having been massaged. "Now that your body has felt that human touch, stay aware of your body and how truly wonderful you can feel with something as simple as a massage. All the more so with lomi lomi, as it is a powerful cleansing and healing massage."

Now, sitting on their stumps around the campfire, Sister says,

> "In most cultures, traditions of healing are sacred and passed down orally. Some of these ancient Hawaiian wisdoms have been lost. In Kemet (ancient Egypt), some of the wisdom was kept on papyrus, some etched on the stone of walls and ceilings in the temples (in Medu Neter, an ancient Egyptian pictographic writing), and sadly, some was lost or destroyed by invaders. Ancient wisdom in Chinese medicine was preserved in the Yellow Emperor's Inner Canon (Huangdi Neijing), a fundamental text for two thousand years.

> "Remember, less than a hundred years ago, it was common to use herbal medicine and all the healing arts during sickness and disease. Only in the last seventy-five years has the medical model for health and wellness changed into a more pharmaceutical norm. This hasn't benefited most people. Today, the US spends the highest proportion of its gross domestic

product on healthcare yet is thirty-seven in performance. Out of thirty-five countries, the US infant mortality rate stands at twenty-nine.

During this week, we have been treating the whole person holistically. We are treating the cause and not just symptoms. You have been reflecting on the issues that concern you. In essence, you have been treating yourself, healing from the inside out—healing your inner self. I am shining the light for you to see more clearly the beauty of your inner self and the power you have to heal yourself.

Regarding evidence-based studies, many such studies, on which the entire industry has based its treatment methods, later were found fraudulent. In general, studies have to meet rigid criteria and exclude many demographics to obtain funding. This creates a homogenous group to the exclusion of a true heterogenic demographic. In these groups, oftentimes there are therapeutic failures with increased side effects.

Sara, Western medicine has made incredible strides for some diseases and illnesses. I know you are proud of Western medicine because that is all you know, but that is not all there is. Be open to the possibilities you are being exposed to here.

There is a study I have known about since the late 1990s that I would like to gently explore here in support of wholeness and healing. It is called the Adverse Childhood Experiences Study (ACE). The study looked at over 17,000 adults, following them over several years. The occurrence of an adverse childhood experience, being defined as abuse, neglect, or family dysfunction, had a significant influence on learning, health, and well-being throughout the lifespan. The likelihood of chronic disease, such as hypertension, diabetes, and cancer, was significantly increased if adverse events had occurred. Disease is dis-ease at a cellular level. These events disrupt neurodevelopment; they cause social, emotional, and cognitive impairment, leading to risky behaviors, and ultimately to disability, disease, and death."

Lew looks up at Sister and says, "So you mean to tell me that if my parents neglected and abused me as a child, it would affect me getting high blood pressure and diabetes and determine how long I live?"

"Yes, Lew," Sister replies, "there are other determinants, but the evidence in this study is compelling."

Lew nods; he quietly reflects on his own son, Solomon, and thinks about providing a better environment for him.

Sister continues.

"The issues, these adverse events, really are in our tissues. Your cells never forget emotional or physical trauma. The memories get trapped in your body as a child. As you grow older, you need to do the hard work of excavating these memories. The point is that these traumas, large or small, are trapped in your tissues, and I have tried to give you some tools to work with them.

"It is not enough to just learn about them and try them out. You have to practice and, when you go home, incorporate these tools into your daily routine. Keep the momentum you have gained. Give attention daily to your mind, body, spirit, and soul. As you have witnessed, small changes can be significant. We heal from the inside out. There is a homunculus, like a small being, on your feet, hands, and ears. All areas of your body are represented and thus can be accessed. A hand or foot massage can do wonders for your weary soul on a stress-filled day. Some of you had a total body massage; others, only your hands and feet. Let me show you what I mean."

Sister beckons the group to gather in more closely around her. She points out the areas they should massage, using her hand and he foot to demonstrate, to address issues in various parts of their bodies. And she shows them the proper touch and motions to use for massage. She gives a short demonstration on each of their hands to give them a feel for depth of touch and the sensation when it is being done.

Then they all gather for their well and lock fingers in a circle. It has been a long, emotional day for them all. The positive energy of their touch, of their human connection forming this circle, gives each of them a bracing sensation, as they ponder what they will take out of the well today.

There can be no keener revelation of a society's soul than the way in which it treats its children.

—Nelson Mandela

Massage Recap

*Anyone wishing to study medicine
must master the art of massage.*

—Hippocrates

Sara—Physician experiencing burnout who is out of touch with herself.

Sister's Solution—Balance and awareness. Tapping the inmost self with honest soul reflection. Giving time for self-care, cultivating self-love and forgiveness. The heart of a healer providing massage and touch can restore life to a sick soul. Granting permission to not know everything of the mind, allowing the heart to *feel* the void.

Massage—Enhances good health. Promotes relaxation; reduces anxiety; improves sleep; reduces muscle tension; lowers blood pressure; improves cardiovascular health; increases range of motion; improves digestive disorders and headaches; enhances exercise performance; decreases arthritic pain; beneficial for fibromyalgia, myofascial pain syndromes, and back pain.

Chapter Six

Yoga

*If you're always trying to be normal, you will
never know how amazing you can be.*

—Maya Angelou

Reiko

Reiko has always enjoyed yoga, practicing it intermittently. She feels like she already knows some of the things Sister has been introducing them to—breathing and silence and massage, now yoga—yet, as Sister is offering them, they feel unique. So, she does not jump to any conclusions about what she does and doesn't know, not since the first day when they had hiked out to the banyan tree and she discovered her deep affinity for the butterflies that had come out to greet her.

Sister has gathered them in this place high up Mauna Kea, toward which they have been hiking all morning. It is not at the summit, which tops out at about 13,000 feet, but they have probably made it to at least 3,000 feet. It is an amazing place, with a sizeable area from which to look out on exhilarating views. And speaking of exhilarating, Reiko also is keen to the energy she senses in returning to this mountain.

They each carried a mat Sister had given them at the start of their hike and are now choosing a spot to place it under the large spreading tree Sister has chosen. They each have an extra towel to fold and put in position to slightly bolster the upper body. They settle into a seated position facing Sister, who is sitting closest to the tree, with her legs gracefully wrapped in a lotus posture. Her hands are relaxed on her knees with her thumbs touching a finger and pointing upward. She sits breathing deeply for a few moments, saying nothing, and they all eventually fall into line with their own breathing, almost entraining to her slow inhalations and exhalations.

Eventually, Sister says softly, "Today, we are going to do a tension-releasing form of yoga, my version of Yoga Nidra. We will also do a restorative yoga." Sister instructs them in a few gentle poses and then says, "Lie back on your mats and relax, like we did when we were doing the breathing exercises."

Sara is flat on her back gazing up at the clouds, listening to Sister's voice flow over her like the pikake-scented oils she had used to massage her the day before. She feels loose and kind of mesmerized as she views the clouds passing overhead, letting them go as easily as she is releasing the thoughts that drift into her mind. This feels good and new. Her mind is calm, and she continues taking long, slow breaths along with the instructions Sister is giving her.

Lew has fallen asleep, and a soft snore is rising from his throat. Even that is not sticking to Sara's notice, as she takes it in, realizes it is, once again, Lew who is creating a slight distraction, and she lets it go, forming an inner smile. This asana, or posture, is about fully letting go.

Nora is so relaxed after a few minutes of remaining in this asana, she finds herself purring like a kitten. No one knows why cats purr, but they do release a gentle rippling vibration from their center when they are content and relaxed, and she feels like her own purring is also a delightful mystery. This sensation is more affirmation for her discovery of the things she needs to keep her life balanced and well.

Ira is in his own world, eyes closed; he is once again in nature, not in a sleeping dream, but waking. He is back in his healing garden, the one he has not yet manifested in the physical world. But it is coming together, almost of its own accord, in his heart, mind, and spirit. He is pleased to have this time to lie down and visit his new happy place.

Reiko feels a gentle wind gliding over her face; there does seems to be more air movement at this elevation. It is enough to bend the trees and she can hear the soft whooshing sounds they are making as the currents flow off them and over her supine body resting on the bolstered mat. She finds herself tuning in closely to sounds, as she keeps her eyes closed. Her awareness is heightened, as she stays open to the positive energy flowing through her. It is pure joy.

Sister's voice continues to come in every now and then, as she speaks and falls silent for intervals, drawing the group into a deeper and deeper state of tranquility. She encourages them to notice what is around and within them, and to be open to sounds, smells, sensations, emotions, thoughts, and to just let these sensations flow over them and welcome what comes next.

After an hour or so, Reiko has really lost track of time. Her thoughts drift back a few years to the sorority social on campus. She'd signed up, but felt uncomfortable in the ethnic clubs, and the business club seemed a bit too nerdy for her. She questioned whether they really accepted her. She would have been the first biracial to pledge. They seemed nice and encouraged her, but she quit. She didn't feel she belonged. They didn't reject her; she rejected herself. Just like in high school. She was tall, tan, black curly hair, almond eyes with epicanthal folds. She'd been told many times she was gorgeous, and she was selected as one of the Cherry Blossom Court for cultural day. She would have become Miss Cherry Blossom, but the committee was not comfortable with her identity—in her heart she knows it to be true.

That certainly wasn't the first time she'd felt this nagging sense of unspoken ill will and exclusion. She just didn't have the courage to keep bolstering herself against it, and so she quit trying. It felt like the recurring tides—every time she had gathered strength to move toward the vast ocean over a wide-open, sunny, sandy beach, telling herself she belonged as much as anyone else, she would find herself in retreat when the inevitable waves started racing up behind her, forcing her to hide.

She suspects a lot of folks would envy her life, seen from a bird's-eye view. Her parents love each other, and she has had all the comforts that money can buy. A warm flush fills her chest as she recalls sitting at the big table in her father's office, crayons in hand, working diligently to stay in the lines and get the pressure just right so her picture would please him enough to put it on his cork board. "I love you, Chichi," she thinks, taking slow, deep breaths.

He would take her to work over the years and proudly introduce her to people who came to his office. She remembers the first time an older woman took a second surprised look at her as she was being introduced, which Reiko couldn't quite figure out. But over time, she got it. Little Reiko could see her own face looking back at her in the mirror, and she had seen no one else with similar features—her light-brown coloring or curly hair—anywhere in Tokyo. Except her mother, but even then, she looked different from Reiko.

Reiko has uncertain memories of her time with her mother's family. She still has not found her emotional center with them. She adores her cousins, and whenever her family would travel to New York, she had such a good time with them. Their hair was as curly as hers, and they had an even darker brown skin tone than her own. But neither of her cousins cared about that stuff at all; they just liked each other.

A sudden image of running around, laughing, and playing with them on the playground, that awful day when she fell off the monkey bars and broke her arm. So much pain! She just wanted her parents to be there, right away, and she cried out to them in Japanese, over and over. She spoke English just fine, but Japanese was more natural to her. She didn't even realize how all the other kids were staring at her, until she calmed down a little. Then, when she became aware of it, she had a sick feeling quite apart from her aching arm. But her cousins, the two of them, got right down with her and stayed close, comforting her until the grown-ups showed up.

She also loves Granny, but that one time she overheard her mother and grandmother having it out always cast a bit of doubt in that direction. She didn't know if Granny had said unkind things, or if she was just telling her mother what others would say. But, boy, her mother let her have it and told Granny no one had better treat her girl any differently than any of her cousins. It was the first time Reiko realized that Granny hadn't wanted her mother to marry her father. It left an odd, tight sensation at the back of her throat that came back anytime this memory flashed into her mind.

And she knows her father's family had not been pleased either. Her grandparents are so quiet, not at all like her New York kin, so you'd have to look carefully to detect it. But look she did, once they got back from that New York visit. That tiff between her mother and Granny got her to wondering whether her Tokyo family had similar feelings.

She eventually asked her older cousin about it, and he just looked at her as if to say, "You've got to be kidding!" and laughed a little, as he brushed by her and walked away. What conclusion could she have drawn, other than neither family had really wanted her to come into the world? Except her mother and father—she had no doubts they had always wanted her, even before she came along.

Still, New York was a lot different from Tokyo. Everyone in New York did not have similar features and a clear set of cultural notions. Quite the opposite. Through most of her childhood, she'd felt that if she could live in New York, maybe her sense of standing out (and not in a good way) would ease up. But over the years, she realized this particular issue would also come up in New York, in a somewhat different way. She'd always dreamed of going to college in the United States, and while she did blend in more at school than she had back home, she did not really fit in.

Nonetheless, the plans her father is making for her are not what she wants. She knows this in her gut. This man he expects her to marry is nice enough, but marriage? Not her choice. As it is, she went to business school to please her father because he had always made it clear he would name her successor to his substantial real estate legacy, and she needed to be worthy. But he also made it clear that there would need to be the "right" man by her side in that endeavor. And, to be frank, he wants her to stay put in Japan. Her becoming a woman of business in his home country, planted within the bonds of marriage would accomplish his wishes.

No matter how clear she has been with herself about not wanting this proffered life, she has not been able to tell him and make him understand. She simply lacks the courage. She can hardly bear the thought of disappointing him. And every time she gives him some wishy-washy comments regarding her feelings on the subject, he just brushes it all away, certain he will get her to come around to his wishes, both for her future in business and marriage.

Reiko continues breathing deeply, following Sister's voice and focusing on letting these thoughts and feelings drift over her. In fact, she is surprised that she is feeling so tranquil, having let her mind run along this track. Such a flow of thoughts generally increases anxiety in her body, but not today.

Sister gently starts bringing them back from their yoga mind. They repeat some gentle stretches and soft poses, then gather up their things to hike back to the house. When they get back to the house, they have some hibiscus tea and fruit, then gather in the yard again on the koa stumps.

Once everyone has settled in, Sister says,

> "I hope you enjoyed the yoga. Yoga means *yoke* or *bind* in Sanskrit. In Kemet, yoga was called Smai Tawi, meaning *union of the two lands*. Yoga has been a practice on Earth for ten thousand years. It a union of body and mind, essentially the binding or the union of your higher self with your lower self. Each of you has an individual consciousness in the way that you perceive your world. But there is the universal consciousness that is far beyond what you can perceive. Yoga is a way to unite your personal consciousness with the universal consciousness, because that is the consciousness that is stable. Universal consciousness never changes; it is all-knowing.

> "Different cultures call it different names, but the differences don't matter because they are all seeking the same thing— to practice a way of uniting the individual with the divine

energy. Christians call it *God*. Buddhists might refer to *cosmic consciousness* or *Buddha-mind*, Taoists call it *the way*. It is all about reaching the ultimate goal of higher enlightenment—the unity of the personal consciousness with the higher consciousness.

"Tapping into the cosmic force will enhance your life in fundamental ways. It will allow you to find better insights within your own mind and to communicate more fully with other people. You will grow to become more self-accepting, sensing the strength and beauty of your inner self. You will ease into a sense of belonging with others, whom you will understand more fully, and whom will find you understandable and worthy of love.

"It is said that the Hawaiian Islands are the chakras of the planet—the Big Island is the heart chakra. There are seven main islands in the Hawaiian chain, each vibrating at a different energy level. They are a part of what is known to be a vortex. That is a high-energy, magnetic, spiritual environment. When you close your eyes, you might be able to appreciate that. It is subtle, but potent, energy. That is why you're here, why you've been drawn to this retreat."

Reiko is fascinated by what Sister has been telling them, and she speaks up suddenly, saying, "Oh, my goodness, I just thought my arms had fallen asleep. They were tingling so."

"Reiko," Sister says, "that is the energy, that is exactly what you were feeling. You were feeling the mana, Reiko. You have opened your spirit and the mountain is responding to your energy. Your channels are open."

"Yes, I feel it!" says Reiko.

"Channels of love," Sister continues, "and forgiveness. By letting go, you give yourself permission to grow and be free from the drama that ensnares others. You are free."

Reiko thinks, "Yes, I am free, free as a butterfly."

Sister falls quiet a moment to let all she has said sink in, and then she says, "All of you have seen butterflies while you were here, in the garden or on the trails. Butterflies are the spirit of reflection and transformation. Indigenous cultures understand the appearance of insects and animals as signs from the spirit world. Be aware of these subtle energies and clues, which can guide you. Many organisms undergo metamorphosis during the final stage—lasting weeks, months, or even years. It is the most difficult stage. Some of you have been cocooning for some time, but now your rebirth is happening."

Reiko's thoughts drift to her grandma (obasan), smiling as Reiko played in Baba's garden. "*Utsukushi cho (beautiful butterfly),*" she would say, pointing and smiling at Reiko, "cho!" Now Reiko knows her baba was right—she is the butterfly, light and free. She has danced to everybody else's beat, but not her own. She has been developing inwardly during this cocoon stage into the person she is destined to become in spirit, mind, and body.

Sister continues, "After the butterfly has emerged from the chrysalis, it waits for its wings to dry before flying."

Sister pauses a moment, and then says, "We'll have lunch shortly, and then you can spend the afternoon as you like. When we gather this evening, on our last day of retreat, we'll be doing a stargazing exercise."

Reiko is feeling satisfied, deeply content, and energized, all at the same time. She is looking forward to the stargazing, and just having the rest of the day to wander around and enjoy the beauty of this place. She feels more solid, like she has built up her fortitude, yet, at the same time she is softer, more open. It feels as if one is supporting the other. She feels like she has room to let herself take some time to explore more fully who this person inside actually is. She has had glimpses of her beauty and strength, and she has come to feel such tenderness for this person inside, she now knows she can be resolute in protecting her, if needed.

Reiko recalls when she arrived at Sister's the first day. She had come early and did some hiking in the area, so it was no big deal to find she had to walk up the hill to the house from the road. She'd been in the area for more than a day and had been outdoors most of that time. She was feeling good and more energetic than she had been before coming to Hawaii. She attributed it to the good ocean air and her inclination for exercise. But as she walked up the drive to Sister's house, she felt inside of her the rightness of coming here. She'd thought of her sudden decision to register for this retreat as kind of quirky and was unsure of whether she should actually come. But the closer she came to her time of arrival, she found her foothold. She is so glad she did. Especially so, after meeting Sister at her front door.

Sister had showed her to her room in a warm and welcoming manner. She then noticed the flower Reiko was holding and asked her if she had picked it on her way to the house. Reiko is sure she turned red, as she felt she had been caught taking something she had no right to. But Sister seemed pleased, almost amused. She took the flower in hand and told her, "Well, this is a naupaka. This flower you chose to carry with you is actually half of a whole. See the blossom; it is one of two varieties. This one grows in the mountains. The other at the beach. Each bears a half blossom that when put together, forms a perfect flower. Of course, there is an ancient legend behind it. I'll tell you about it later in the week."

Sister did tell her the rest of the story on the first day while they were hiking. It involves lovers who were separated and turned into flowers, and who can only be joined when they have been picked.

Reiko needs time to take all this in and come to terms with herself more fully. But that is okay. She feels capable of it now, whereas when she came here, she was not so sure of anything. Then, she had sensed she could be pulled off her own center in one direction or another. In particular, she'd had a fear of going home and falling under too much influence of her parents, afraid of where that might lead. Now, not so much. She loves them, and she needs them. But she needs herself even more. And that is who she will need to remain true to.

She is coming to believe she can do that—she will do that. At last, she is excited about her potential, rather than fearful, and she is keenly aware this fresh sense of self-acceptance is the catalyst. Bolstered by an infusion of intestinal fortitude, Reiko is amazed and joyful to feel so newly empowered.

"I can do this. My wings are a little damp, but I will fly. I will just be fine."

#   #   #

Sister carves out some time for herself in the course of the afternoon. She has planned for everyone to have time to themselves today. By this point in the week, she finds the solo time is as welcome for her as for any of them. She has been looking in on them intermittently and staying generally aware of how they are spending their afternoon, but now she leaves herself an hour or so before it will be time to start dinner. She settles into the koa rocker in her room and closes her eyes.

The energy of this group is pleasing, and she feels particularly close to them, even more so than with other groups. She cannot put her finger on any reason, but she is enjoying it. She feels a little emotional knowing the week soon will come to an end. They each have something so special about them, a quality of energy, vulnerability, and dedication to service, to higher ideals. Quite wonderful. And yet, challenging, particularly Lew and Sara. They have been draining, coming for help, yet so resistant to what she has to teach. All the more reason why they needed to come here.

She takes a deep breath and thinks of her family. She feels some sadness at not having them nearby, but, as always, she meditates and prays and continues to connect using her mana to bless and heal. She is grateful for this group with her today, with whom she is able to connect—giving to and receiving from them. In their presence, she is beginning to wonder whether it might be time for her to follow her own advice and find a way to reframe some of her own life decisions, to find a way to reconnect.

# # #

They have a late dinner and take time to talk to one another around the table afterward. Ira is talking about his ideas for starting a new business when he returns home and explaining the great pleasure he's found in Sister's gardens. He invites them all to watch for his new enterprise within the next two or three years. He will have a lot of work to do, getting his healing gardens planted, and finding the right people to come in and help him with that.

Nora tells them about her little girls and has some cute stories, especially about her youngest, Kayla, whom she describes as a *firecracker*. She mentions she has been homeschooling them for a few years now and is thinking it might be time to enroll them in school and see how that goes. Two of her girls are quite social, and they are all sharp and should do well. "I'm seeing how I've maybe taken on more than I need to, and how I need to carve out some time for myself," she says. She seems more relaxed than a few days ago, when the threads of her anxiety had still been clinging to her.

Reiko says to Nora, almost shyly, "You're lucky to have your family. It's all in place for you. Your beautiful daughters, and, with your education, you can go back to work eventually, if you like. I think I was a little envious of you, and maybe I still am." Reiko laughs a little and continues, "But I see now that it must be hard to keep up with so much every day. My life is fairly quiet and calm compared to yours. I spend a lot of time doing the things I enjoy, like hiking. So, I guess I've got it good."

Nora looks at Reiko a moment, and then smiles. "Yeah, well, right back at you. I think I've been a little envious of your life. Probably for similar reasons. You're young and unencumbered right now. You can do whatever you want. Well, I know it's not that easy, even so, we all have something to deal with, obstacles that we have to learn to work through."

Nora hasn't realized she'd been feeling that way until she says those words to Reiko. She has been finding her a little annoying all week, without being able to put her finger on the reason. She has been telling herself she finds her immature. Judging her. But the truth is Nora is envious. Young and full of energy and strength and having her whole life ahead of her to decide whatever she wants to do.

Nora had been like that once, then she just fell into married life. And she's had trouble coping ever since. She is so glad that Reiko spoke up like that. She wouldn't want to have left without understanding the dynamic they've fallen into almost from the start of the week. She puts her hand on Reiko's arm, and says, "Thanks, Reiko, for saying all that. You have a lot of insight into people."

Reiko looks a little startled by her comment. But she's pleased.

The evening sky is quickly transforming into a night sky, when they gather outside. The heavens gradually darken and brighten, all at the same time. Thousands of points of light shine out in a way that none of them has seen before this week, except Lew and Uncle. Uncle always appreciated the stars for their sublime presence but hasn't taken time to study them. Lew has seen skies like that while still in the service, stationed in far-off reaches of the world. But he never valued them, having his attention fixated on more immediate situations that required his constant attention.

Lew focuses on the twinkling stars now. They are everywhere, like sand grains on the beach. "Twinkle, twinkle, little star," he hums softly. The expansiveness of it all helps him breathe a little deeper. *The universe, life is amazing. The creator of all this grandness must have a greater plan for me. I will remind myself to look for the answers,* he thinks with resolve.

Here, tonight, they are all relaxed and taking in the vast beauty laid out before them like an opened gift. After a time of silence, Sister says,

> "Hawaiians in ancient times navigated the oceans. They accomplished this amazing feat by navigating using the stars

alone. Hōkūle'a traveled the oceans all over the world, using ancient methods. No fancy equipment, nothing modern. Hōkūle'a returned after three years of world travel. The ancients used the stars of Orion's Belt as the basis for their charting. Actually, the great pyramids, Khafre, Khufu, and Menkaure, are lined up with Orion's Belt. The meaning of the stars has fascinated civilizations from ancient times. The stars are always there, and to tap into their guidance, you simply need to become aware of them. It is a powerful thing to do in life.

"Stars can be our guides to illuminate our path, gods for us to revere, or compasses to show us the way. Each of you must search your soul for the truth and revelation that resides in your DNA deep inside."

Sitting around a crackling campfire and embracing the vast, brilliant world overhead, which feels just a little bit more intimate than it had before today, all of them are glad to extend the time of their gathering on this serene last night together.

Your heart knows the way. Run in that direction.

—Rumi

Yoga Recap

Yoga is not about touching your toes.
It is what you learn on the way down.

—Jigar Gor

Reiko—Young woman enmeshed in naïveté and frustration in dealing with challenges of her biracial identity, as she heads out on the road of adult life.

Sister's Solution—Self-reflection and appreciation of her duality, embracing the yin/yang of yoga to balance her life.

Yoga—Improves mental health problems: depression, anxiety, insomnia, and addiction. Increases bliss and pleasure, decreases fear and rage, increases pleasure sensations. Improves physical and emotional well-being, flexibility, and posture; loosens muscles; decreases pain; builds muscle mass; maintains strength, protects against arthritis. Improves cardiovascular function, heart health, blood flow, and lymphatic drainage; regulates adrenal gland function; lowers cortisol levels; increases serotonin levels; decreases blood pressure. Improves balance; promotes breathing and lung function.

Chapter Seven

Farewell

Give the ones you love wings to fly, roots to come back and reasons to stay.

—Dalai Lama XIV

"It is important that you give something to the island, and that you take something away," Sister says, looking around the group, making eye contact with each of them. Everyone has gathered outside in their morning circle, having packed their belongings and shared a satisfying meal together. Everyone had risen early and helped Sister prepare a delicious breakfast of soursop, mango, papaya, taro bread with ginger, and hibiscus tea to celebrate their last day together. Now they have gathered on the stumps for the last time before heading off to return to their lives after this reprieve.

Ira speaks up, "Hey, Sister, I thought that was kapu. Removing something? I heard that was a bad thing."

Nora chimes in, "Yeah, I heard people say they had back luck if they took a lava rock, or something like that, from the island.

"Wait a minute. Wait a minute," Sister replies. "Yes, yes, it is kapu to remove material things that belong to Mother Nature. Natural artifacts belong to the universe. Don't remove stones or other things because you want to keep them in place for more people to enjoy." Sisters smiles a little and adds, "The goddess Pele might have a penchant for punishing pilferers, and many stories do address that. You know that it's common sense not to steal, so you only take that which belongs to you, that which is in your heart."

Sister bends and picks up a leaf from the grass and holds it up. "You can give something by choosing a leaf, or use a piece of stone or sea glass, or whatever works for you. I want you to write or etch on it your name, or a word, or something that symbolizes you or something significant to you. But it is important that you leave it, as it will become part of the art that decorates my home. Thus, each of you will leave part of yourself here.

"That box I presented to you on our first day together is your toolbox. It will keep you safe. The things you carry in it will help you handle your day-to-day challenges. Let me explain."

Sister pauses, looking around her at their attentive faces arranged in a loose circle where they are occupying the koa stumps, and then says, "So, these lessons you have learned on this island, you will keep with you. Keep these safe in your box. The most valuable things are the memories you take with you. They can become embedded in your hearts and give you peace as you touch them in your travels.

"In the course of our time together, you learned about nutrition of the heart, about primary and secondary nutrition. You also learned about maat, about being balanced and about how your heart would be weighed to determine whether it was light enough, thus virtuous, to permit entry into a happy afterlife. Guilt, worry, regret, anger, sadness—all these burden your heart; all these increase cortisol, increase inflammation, causing illness and disease. Put nutrition into your box."

Sister turns her head to Sara. "Sara, you learned about touch. I just want you and Lew," she says turning to Lew to include him in her comments, "to realize how much you two have in common. It is about acceptance through love, and not so much about how to be with others, but yourself. You both took a vow of allegiance. Sara, you took an allegiance to medicine. Lew, you took an allegiance to the military. But your first allegiance needs to be to yourself."

Sara and Lew are listening closely to Sister, and both seem a little perplexed. But they are open to hearing what she has to say, having come to trust her wisdom.

"During the process of providing your service—you, Sara, in service to medicine and you, Lew, in service to your country in the military—you might have become disenchanted. That disenchantment can present itself as anxiety, compassion fatigue, PTSD, or burnout—each is just one point on the same line. I think you both probably have a lot of truth and morality in your hearts. It hurts to sin against yourself, and so I think you might have been looking for answers, for ways to shield yourself from some of that injury and pain.

"Moral injury—that is what this kind of injury has been called. I call it 'heart hurt,'" Sister continues. "It is when you are called to do something that is against your will or conscience—a moral transgression that causes shame. So, for you, Lew, who wanted to enter the ministry at one time, and then you ended up on the battlefield, killing. Of course, that is an attack on your own soul and spirit, and your own morality. That must have been all the more challenging for you, because you were a man of faith. You are a man of faith. It is essential for you to realize that it wasn't your fault. Not only had you been commanded to do so, but had you failed at it, you would also have been killed."

Lew is fully attentive to Sister, with his eyes locked on her face. He is still for a change and leaning toward her with his forearms leaning on his thighs. He says nothing. It is unclear how he is responding at this point. Someone watching him might venture a guess that he would soon pop off in anger, or dismiss her words with disdain, or fully absorb those words and start a new path for himself, any of them could turn out to be so, given how inscrutable he looks in the moment.

"So, you, Sara, wanted to be a healer, a doctor, to help people, yet you know in your heart that many of the prescription medicines you're giving are treating the symptoms but not the causes. And the side effects can be life-threatening. That doesn't cure anything. Rather than get better, patients seem to get worse. And in the middle of all that, you are not able to spend the time you would like with your patients.

You used to enjoy talking with your patients, learning about their stories, finding out more about their families. Now you're under production pressure and have about fifteen minutes to spend with each of them, and if you spend more time, you're penalized, and it has an impact on your livelihood. Not meeting these metrics affects your income and your privileges. You stay late after hours trying to catch up, missing important sporting activities and engagements with your children. That is not how you envisioned your life in medicine years ago when you dreamed of becoming a doctor. I know you have a healing heart for your patients. Remember the healing touch you received. Now you know that just a simple touch or a hand on the shoulder can go a long way."

Sister falls silent for a moment to let her words settle. "So, you end up feeling like a cog in the wheel. You are ensconced in the middle of the system, and, frankly, I think you would be happier if you were to find your own place, away from there, where you could take care of your patients and engage in the healing work that's truly in your heart. It is a difficult choice. It might affect your bottom line but overall it will improve the quality of your life, which is priceless." Sara sits silently, watching Sister closely, waiting to hear what else she will say about this.

Sister continues, "Just like you, Lew. There is also an epidemic with soldiers. The system is changing, but there is a high rate of suicide among soldiers who have come back from the Iraqi and Afghani campaigns. The rate is about one soldier per day. While the system is changing, it is not evolving quickly enough to get our soldiers the help they need and the tools that can enable them to heal the mind, body, and spirit. Beforehand, the doctors had been just handing out medication, not treating veterans fairly, and making access to care nearly impossible.

"Sara, the statistics are similar for physicians. The burnout rate across most specialties for physicians is about fifty percent. And the suicide rate among physicians is about the same as for soldiers—more than one each day. That's almost four hundred every year. Suicide is the leading cause of death among physicians. That's the dirty little secret! So, Sara and Lew, you have more in common than you might believe."

Sister leans back a little, as she had been focused intently on Sara and Lew, and now she is taking in the overall group. "The tools you have learned here will help heal the mind, the body, and the spirit. There is space to run. There is space to be free. You're free from judgment, eating organic foods and nutritional herbs, letting Mother Nature heal you, getting love and camaraderie from one another. Opening yourselves to receive the healing touch of lomi lomi. Self-reflection, transparency, and honesty with yourselves. These are the things that will heal you, no matter the cause. Put movement in your box, Lew. Put massage in your box, Sara.

"Each of you has a story. You need to share your stories. In the sharing of your stories, being able to get that all into the open and out of your system, you will be able to release those thoughts, and that will help you heal. You need to work and till your gardens. The answers are all in the soil. But the soul is the soil that we till for everlasting peace and a good life. That is what I want for each of you."

She looks at Lew. "The system is broken, Lew, but you can be part of the change. Charge up the hill of change! You are articulate and intelligent. Use your gifts to organize and get the funding to help yourself and your battle buddies. Tell your story as only you can. You know that cannabis helps with your symptoms better than any of the other medications you have tried. You know counseling works, and especially when it is given by others who have served, because it provides a sense of safety, trust, and kinship. You have a heart for service, Lew. Let it serve you by helping others. It will be therapeutic for you."

Sister looks at Ira, and says, "Uncle, you are so knowledgeable about the land, the aina. And I know that you will heal. I want you to consider coming back. We could use some help around here with the garden and crops. I want to use your store of knowledge and wisdom about farming to expand our crops. You have a gift with the soil and this type of work will heal your heart."

Uncle looks a little humbled and enormously pleased. He had planned to ask Sister for the opportunity to return for her wisdom, and here she was offering him what he needed and asking him, with deep respect, to share what he had to offer.

He says softly, "Maybe the universe knows best in pointing me in this direction. If my boys, Chuck and Willie, hadn't done what they did, I would never have come here to you, Sister. I would never have been to this incredible place and met these wonderful people, and I would never have learned what you've been teaching me here this past week."

Sister looks pleased at Uncle Ira's response and nods at him with a smile. Then, she looks at Nora and asks her how the week has been for her. She notices that Nora has placed a hibiscus snugly behind her ear.

Nora replies, "You know what? I have some challenges I need to address with my husband when I get home. We need to make some changes, and I need to let him know what we need to make our marriage work. We need to figure that out together. I am going to volunteer and get back to doing some of the things that I enjoy, and just make space to do the things I need to nurture myself. I haven't felt this centered in an awfully long time. I'm not letting that go, now that I know the path to take me there. I also know that the things that bring me peace and happiness are my family. So, I'm going to focus more on me. If I'm happy and take care of myself, then I will be more available and less resentful."

Sister nods with an affirming smile, and says, "Well, it doesn't have to be either/or. You can have a happy family and be happy. With better balance, you won't build up resentment in your heart, and your children will appreciate you more. Parenting is challenging, but, in many ways, less is more. Letting children learn from their own mistakes builds their confidence and strength. Put mindfulness in your box."

Nora laughs and say, "It's only been one week, and I got a complete makeover. Now this is retail therapy. An incredible return on my investment."

Sister looks at Reiko.

Reiko pipes up, "I've come away with a firmer sense of myself this week. I'm okay with me now. I don't have to fit into any mold. I thought I did, but I've become more aware of me as me. I am more self-aware and self-accepting, and, frankly, I'm okay with that. I kind of like it." She smiles confidently. She seems radiant, certainly more relaxed than when they'd met her, a few days before.

Reiko has come into her awareness with a new sense of self-confidence. She is neither refined nor polished, but she understands her own power, and that inner knowledge, in itself, is empowering. She is complete within herself, comfortable and content with who she is becoming. She had an epiphany during her meditation, realizing she does not need to be or do anything special to fit in. Living in the now is enough. The world—both the yin and the yang—are within and need to be embraced. All of us are duality, and expressions of our individual creativity are unique. Looking in the mirror of her soul, she is whole and full. Satisfied with self-love. Able to accept her differences and embrace them in others.

Sister places her hand over Reiko's for a moment, and says, "Reiko, you can go anywhere and do anything because that's who you are. What you are looking for, you already have. Put yoga in your box."

Sister then looks over at Sara, and says, "Sara, thank you for sharing your story about your grandmother this morning at breakfast. As children we have elaborate imagination and creativity. We tell ourselves stories that might or might not be true. We hold these stories in our hearts, and they become our truth. You know your grandmother died, not because you fell on her, but because her disease had run its course. Most likely, you were her favorite, and she was hanging on to see your sparkling eyes and receive your sweet kiss one more time.

"We have to frame these childhood experiences differently. This week, we had an opportunity to look at the past, at our memories, and we need to reframe them with our new awareness, with our new truth. And that is the real farming you need to do, digging in your soul, tilling the land of your soul, and the harvest will be bountiful, if the work has been done."

Sister stands, steps toward Sara, and gives her a hug. A full twelve-second hug as on the first day, only this time, she is not the only one hugging. Today, Sara leans warmly into Sister's embrace and encircles her with her arms. Instead of waiting for Sister to complete the circle, the rest of the group look around at one another and start leaning into each other with hugs, each at least as long as Sister's famous hugs. Sister has hugged each of them, and they stand there, basking in the warmth and tingle of the energy they have exchanged, waiting for Sister to say something.

Sister says, "huli huli," and they all say, "huli huli," with bright smiles, as they turn over their bowls. Sister sees the radiance of each soul before her. Light has filled each heart, and so the journey continues. Sister steps up to embrace each of them once again, and to give them her parting message.

Sister embraces Sara, heart to heart, to give and receive the gift of love, the only true healing power of the universe. Sister whispers in her ear, "Touch, the healing power of touch is in your hands."

She moves on to Lew, and after embracing him warmly, she whispers, "Lew, movement. The exercise will keep you fit, and your thoughts will run away, not with you. They will lose their power over you. It was not your fault, Lew. Your heart is golden. Forgive yourself, you owe it to your soul."

To Nora, she says softly in her ear, after hugging her, "Nora, meditation and mindfulness will keep you grounded. And buckle your own seatbelt first, sweetie. Honor yourself, and, by taking care of yourself, you'll be better able to take care of your family."

After hugging Uncle Ira, she whispers, "Uncle, nutrition will keep you on track. Remember to feed your soul. That is the greatest gift you can give, not only to yourself but also to your community."

Sister embraces Reiko and whispers, "Reiko, you have accepted yourself, and, by doing so, you allow others to embrace you. The key to your best life is balance. As above, so below. Both parts of you make you whole. Embrace it all."

Stepping back, Sister tells the group in a deep voice that reveals how heartfelt her words are, "Each of you reminds me of some aspect of my life, or a person in my life. I feel we have a connection that extends beyond recognition—a soul connection. We all have problems and troubles and secrets. I came here many years ago to dig into my own soil, my own soul, and to plant the seeds of happiness and health. I have been moved and honored to share what I have learned with you. No longer are these things secrets to you, but they are now a part of who you are. Now, in this sharing, we are one. I have been a cairn to you to point you in a new direction on a new path in your life. There will be others to assist you on your journey. Keep your heart light and your eyes open."

# # #

As they wander to the porch to pick up their bags, Uncle Ira says, "Hey, ladies, I know you need a ride to the airport. I drove here in my truck and would be happy to give you a lift." Smiling broadly, they all accept with enthusiasm. They turn to head toward his truck, parked outside the stone fence, and Uncle Ira turns to Lew and says, "Hey, man, come on. Jump in, and I can drive you where you need to go."

Lew had started heading toward the road and stops to look at Uncle. "Naw, thanks anyway, Uncle. You know I like to run. I like the fresh air. I'm gonna be okay. I'll walk down the hill. Got a lot on my mind, and there's something in particular I really need to do."

Uncle Ira walks over to Lew and says, "Well, okay, man." Uncle gives him a handshake, but then both men pull in close and give each other an earnest hug. Yes, twelve seconds. And Lew heads off, as Uncle Ira and the women head to his truck.

As they walk, everyone keeps turning intermittently and waving at Sister who is standing on the porch watching them leave. Sister's eyes are as full as her heart, and each time someone turns to wave at her, she returns their wave with a slow, wide movement of her whole arm. Once they are all out of view, Sister takes a deep breath and heads back into the kitchen. She had told the group to just leave the dishes that morning, so everyone could stay on schedule for their travel plans. Now she starts washing dishes at the sink and wiping down counters. She will have a day to herself, and then she will start receiving new guests to the retreat planned for the upcoming week. She thinks, *What a good life I have.*

# # #

Lew watches the truck pull past him, moving toward the main road with all its occupants waving at him wildly. He returns their waves and feels a brief flush of sadness wash over him. He had come to feel close to each of them in his way, and what Sister said about Sara that morning has made him think. It has the ring of truth. This point of view Sister explained about them having a lot in common has piqued his curiosity, given how all week Sara seems to have tripped his wires over his medical stuff. He feels there might be more to explore; maybe their paths will cross again on this journey called life.

As he walks, taking in the breathtaking views and breathing the sweet air deeply, he feels energized. It's not about anxiety anymore. He feels peaceful, and an odd sensation rises in his center—pure happiness. He's made a good start this week, he thinks, and is glad deep down that he has come here. Sister has the real stuff to offer, and he feels some hope he can make good on what she has given him.

But first things first. Lew digs into his pocket to retrieve his wallet and cell phone, which have been put away during his time at the retreat— one of Sister's ground rules. He fishes out a folded, crumpled piece of paper from his wallet. He stops in place and turns on his phone as he studies the number, which has become a little faded with time. "Oh, wow," Lew says, "it's an 808 area code. Cool." He takes a deep breath and enters the number.

Reception for cell phones is not great on this part of the Big Island, he knows. He had tried to make some calls when he first arrived. But he can't wait and wants to make the call as soon as possible, now that he has finally gotten himself to this point.

# # #

Sister's phone rings a few times before she can get to it, as she has been puttering about and left it in the bedroom. "Yes, aloha," she says, pressing the button after the fifth ring, catching it in time.

"Is this Lucinda Luvenia?" A warm, familiar male voice inquires and stops her short. She swallows hard, pausing for a long moment, before responding. She hasn't heard that name in years.

"Yes, this is," she says slowly.

"Hi. My name is Lew. I'm your son."

The tears Sister had managed to dry as her guests were leaving come flooding back in a rush, and she drops into her chair, crying and laughing all at the same time. She manages to say, "Lew! Son! Come on back to the house."

Remember that the best relationship is one in which your love for each other exceeds your need for each other.

—Dalai Lama XIV

Note from the Author

Kimberly R. Kelley, MD, MBA
Founder, Director of Core Wellness Hawaii

Mana is a term in Polynesian and Hawaiian culture that refers to a power and energy that lives within all of us. It's the energy we have from birth, which is available to guide us to our greatest potential. Realizing this strength takes place on a road during the journey called life. The road can be meandering, hopeful, challenging, happy, hilly, muddy, narrow, green, windy, sad, joyful, serene, beautiful, and silent. This book tells the stories of five people searching for mana.

I am an anesthesiologist in a hospital in Honolulu, but I wrote this book because I believe in an integrative, holistic approach to healing, applying medical knowledge and empowering individuals to find personal wholeness and wellness through mind, body, spirit, and Mother Earth. This can lead all of us on the road to mana.

I consider myself a "healer by heart, a physician by trade." Besides being an anesthesiologist, I'm also a medical acupuncturist, specializing in anesthesia, acute/chronic pain management, and medical simulation. I received my medical training at Wright State University, Dayton, Ohio. My vast experience in private practice and in the military arena have colored my view of medicine and healing, both in the operating room and beyond.

This is a story about the potency of the healing practices I have come to believe are essential in living a life of wholeness and joy. I chose to present this vital information in the form of a story, because stories are the most fundamental way through which humans understand our place in the world, relying on their power to inform and move us, as we have since ancient times. Through the stories of five people who need healing from common life experiences, I present a path of renewal through five practices: movement, nutrition, mindfulness/ meditation, massage, and yoga.

I invite you consider whether the kind of experience presented in this book through the stories of Sister, Lew, Sara, Nora, Uncle Ira, and Reiko might be what you are looking for at this time in your life. Our vision at Core Wellness Hawaii is healing the inner self by empowering personal wholeness and wellness through the core connection of mind, body, and spirit. We provide a safe and emotionally secure space in a serene tropical locale to allow personal growth and exploration. Our programs provide sustainable transformation by engaging the senses and encouraging self-exploration in nature.

Invitation

You are on the right path.
Discover more! Sign up for a retreat
or workshop today.

Visit our website at
https://corewellnesshawaii.com/ to learn more.

**Feel free to connect and let me
know what you thought of this book.
I would love to hear from you.**

Appendix

Essentials for the Road to Mana Hike

1. Movement

Without mental health there can be no true physical health.

—Dr. Brock Chisholm, World Health Organization

Lew—Physically fit, but emotionally unhealthy.

Sister's Solution—Nonpharmacologic treatments: exercise, focused physical activities (horseback riding, canoeing, hiking), herbal support, and plant-based medicine.

Exercise—Positive effect on depression, anxiety, stress, and PTSD. It can predict morbidity and mortality by affecting weight loss and glucose control. Exercise promotes bone health and mental health and increases immunologic factors. Insufficient exercise results in increased rates of cardiovascular disease and all-cause mortality. Not only can a physically active lifestyle reduce mortality and prevent many chronic diseases, such as hypertension, diabetes, stroke, and cancer, it can promote healthy cognitive and psychosocial function.

2. Nutrition

A merry heart does good, like medicine,
But a broken spirit dries the bones.

—Proverbs 17:22 NKJV

Uncle Ira—Broken heart of unforgivingess and grief.

Sister's Solution—Primary nutrition and secondary nutrition. Ira began to understand how to nourish his soul with happiness, relationships, and love, and learns to fuel his body with the most natural source of organic herbs, fruits, and vegetables from Mother Earth.

Nutrition—Promotes heart health, improves mental clarity, and decreases chronic illness. Diet quality affects mental health brain plasticity. Diet during early life is linked to mental health outcomes in children. Manipulation of the diet directly affects cardiovascular health and heart disease.

3. Mindfulness/Meditation

The best way to capture moments is to pay attention. This is how we cultivate mindfulness.

—Jon Kabat-Zinn

Nora—Lost herself in the midst of motherhood.

Sister's Solution—Self-reflection, work on the breath, meaning of Hawaii, silent meditation.

Mindfulness—Reduces anxiety, reduces implicit age and race bias, might prevent and treat depression, increases body satisfaction, improves cognition, helps the brain stay focused with less distraction. Yoga and meditation practices exert positive influence on addictive behaviors.

4. Massage

Anyone wishing to study medicine
must master the art of massage.

—Hippocrates

Sara—Physician experiencing burnout who is out of touch with herself.

Sister's Solution—Balance and awareness. Tapping the inmost self with honest soul reflection. Giving time for self-care, cultivating self-love and forgiveness. The heart of a healer providing massage and touch can restore life to a sick soul. Granting permission to not know everything of the mind, allowing the heart to *feel* the void.

Massage—Enhances good health. Promotes relaxation; reduces anxiety; improves sleep; reduces muscle tension; lowers blood pressure; improves cardiovascular health; increases range of motion; improves digestive disorders and headaches; enhances exercise performance; decreases arthritic pain; beneficial for fibromyalgia, myofascial pain syndromes, and back pain.

5. Yoga

*Yoga is not about touching your toes. It is
what you learn on the way down.*

—Jigar Gor

Reiko—Young woman enmeshed in naïveté and frustration in dealing with challenges of her biracial identity, as she heads out on the road of adult life.

Sister's Solution—Self-reflection and appreciation of her duality, embracing the yin/yang of yoga to balance her life.

Yoga—Improves mental health problems: depression, anxiety, insomnia, and addiction. Increases bliss and pleasure, decreases fear and rage, increases pleasure sensations. Improves physical and emotional well-being, flexibility, and posture; loosens muscles; decreases pain; builds muscle mass; maintains strength, protects against arthritis. Improves cardiovascular function, heart health, blood flow, and lymphatic drainage; regulates adrenal gland function; lowers cortisol levels; increases serotonin levels; decreases blood pressure. Improves balance; promotes breathing and lung function.

Notes and Suggested Reading

This is a list of resources I have used in writing this book. It is not a complete list of the reading I have done in forming my ideas, but I provide it to point the way to additional resources, which address the underlying concepts presented in this book and in grateful recognition of the valuable insights of these authors.

Introduction

1. "Mana Road," Dangerous Roads (website), accessed May 11, 2018, http://www.dangerousroads.org/north-america/usa/7300-mana-road.html.

2. Derek Paiva, "The Brilliant Beauty of Mauna Kea's Little-Traveled Mana Road," Hawaii Magazine (website), April 24, 2017, accessed May 11, 2018, https://www.hawaiimagazine.com/content/breathtaking-beauty-mauna -keas-little-traveled-mana-road.

Chapter One—Awareness

3. Alaya DeNoyelles, "The Bowl of Light," The Sovereignty of Love (website), accessed May 8, 2018, http://www.sovereigntyoflove.com/the-book/ introduction-the-bowl-of-light/.

4. Hank Wesselman, PhD, "The Bowl of Light: Ancestral Wisdom from a Hawaiian Shaman," Shared Wisdom (website), accessed May 8, 2018, http://www.sharedwisdom.com/product/bowl-light-ancestral-wisdom -hawaiian-shaman.

5. Emily Seymour, "The Bowl of Light," Mind Body Mandala (website), June 14, 2012, accessed May 8, 2018, http://www.mindbodymandala.com/mind -body-mandala/the-bowl-of-light/.

Chapter Two—Movement (Lew)

6. "The History of the Banyan Tree in Hawaii," Hawaii Aloha Travel (website), accessed May 8, 2018, https://www.hawaii-aloha.com/blog/2014/.../the -history-of-the-banyan-tree-hawaii/.

7. "Banyan," Wikipedia, The Free Encyclopedia (website), accessed May 8, 2018, https://en.wikipedia.org/wiki/Banyan.

8. K. A. Babson, A. J. Heinz, G. Ramirez, M. Puckett, J. G. Irons, M. O. Bonn-Miller, S. H. Woodward, "The Interactive Role of Exercise and Sleep on Veteran Recovery from Symptoms of PTSD, *Mental Health and Physical Activity 8*, Elsevier (March 2015) https://pdfs.semanticscholar.org /7c53/186737343361a5cd8a20b272b3596463ef4e.pdf.

9. Michael Tam, "The History of Hawaiian Koa Wood: A True Story," Martin & MacArthur (website), September 30, 2014, accessed May 8, 2018, https:// martinandmacarthur.com/blogs/.../the-history-of-hawaiian-koa-wood-a-true-story.

Chapter Three—Nutrition (Uncle Ira)

10. "Noni," *National Center for Complementary and Integrative Health* (website), September 2016, accessed May 8, 2018, https://nccih.nih.gov/health/noni.

11. Library of Congress Aesop Fables—Read.gov (website), accessed May 8, 2018, http://www.read.gov/aesop/001.html.

12. "Afrikan Holistic Health," The Afrikan Center of Well Being, Inc. (website), accessed May 8, 2018, http://www.acwbinc.org/icm.html.

13. "Why 'Primary Food' Is Integrative Nutrition's Key to Health and Happiness," Integrative Nutrition (website), August 29, 2016, accessed May 8, 2018, https://www.integrativenutrition.com/blog/2016/08/why-primary-food-is-integrative-nutrition-s-key-to-health-and-happiness.

14. "The Goddess Maat, The Maat," Osirisnet (website), accessed May 8, 2018, https://osirisnet.net/dieux/maat/e_maat.htm.

15. Joshua J. Mark, "Ma'at," Ancient History Encyclopedia (website), September 15, 2016, accessed May 8, 2018, https://www.ancient.eu/Ma'at/.

16. Zach Royer, "The 52 Supernatural Places on Hawaii Islands," 52 Perfect Days (website), October 25, 2014, accessed May 8, 2018, https://52perfectdays. com/hawaii/52-supernatural-places-hawaii-

17. "Wisdom of the Ancient Sages," Deep Spirits (website), accessed May 8, 2018, http://www.deepspirits.com/ancient-sages/imhotep/.

Chapter Four—Mindfulness/Meditation (Nora)

18. See note 7 above.

19. "Ha: The Breath of Life," Hawaii Aloha Travel (website), accessed May 8, 2018, https://www.hawaii-aloha.com/blog/2012/04/16/ha-the-breath-of-life/.

20. "Meditation HA Breathing," Ancient Huna.com (website), accessed May 9, 2018, http://www.ancienthuna.com/ha_breathing.htm.

21. "Green Sea Turtle," Wikipedia, The Free Encyclopedia (website), accessed May 9, 2018, https://en.wikipedia.org/wiki/Green_sea_turtle.

22. Jagad Guru Siddhaswarupananda, "The Deeper Meaning of Meditation," Yoga Wisdom (website), December 4, 2016, accessed May 9, 2018, http://wisdom.yoga/deeper-meaning-meditation/.

23. "Heiau," Aloha Condos & Homes (website), accessed May 9, 2018, http://www.alohacondos.com/travel/hawaii/heiau/.

24. The Flower Expert (website), accessed May 9, 2018, https://www.theflowerexpert.com/content/aboutflowers/.../hawaii-state-flowers.

Chapter Five—Massage (Sara)

25. Ilza Veith (Translator), *Medical Classics: The Yellow Emperor's Classic of Internal Medicine* (Oakland: University of California Press, 1975).

26. James Curran (Reviewer), "The Yellow Emperor's Classic of Internal Medicine," US National Library of Medicine National Institutes of Health, BMJ (website), April 5, 2008, accessed May 9, 2018, https://www.ncbi.nlm.nih.gov/pmc/articles/PMC2287209/.

27. E. A. Wallis Budge (Translator), "Papyrus of Ani; Egyptian Book of the Dead [Budge]," University of Pennsylvania-African Studies Center (website), March 3, 1994, accessed May 9, 2018, http://www.africa.upenn.edu/Books/Papyrus_Ani.html.

28. "Adverse Childhood Experiences," SAMHSA (Website), last updated Sept 5, 2017, accessed May 9, 2018, https://www.samhsa.gov/capt/practicing -effective-prevention/prevention-behavioral-health/adverse-childhood -experiences

29. Maulana Karenga, *The Book of Coming Forth by Day: The Ethics of the Declarations of Innocence* (University of Sankore Press, 1990).

30. Tracey Lakainapali, "Hawaiian Lomi Lomi Massage," Aloha International (website), accessed May 9, 2018, https://www.huna.org/html/lomilomi.html.

Chapter Six—Yoga (Reiko)

31. "What Is Kemetic YogaTM?" Yogaskills Kemetic Yoga (website), accessed May 9, 2018, www.kemeticyoga.com/what-is-kemetic-yoga.

32. Brian Handwerk, "Pyramids at Giza," National Geographic (website), accessed May 9, 2018, https://www.nationalgeographic.com/archaeology-and-history/archaeology/giza-pyramids/.

33. Vic Warren, "The Legend of the NapaukaFlower," Vic Warren: The Art of Adventure (website), accessed May 9, 2018, https://www.vicwarren.com/the-legend-of-the-naupaka-flower.

34. "The Story of Hōkūleʻa," Polynesian Voyaging Society (website), accessed May 9, 2018, www.hokulea.com/voyages/our-story/.

35. "The Beautiful Way Hawaiian Culture Embraces a Particular Kind of Transgender Identity," Huffpost (website), updated December 6, 2017, accessed May 10, 2018, https://www.huffingtonpost.com/2015/04/28/hawaiian-culture-transgender_n_7158130.html.

36. Sarah Wells, "Ancient Wisdom—Sacred Alignment and the Constellation of Orion (website), January 1, 2018, https://blog.pachamama.org/ancient -wisdom-sacred-alignment-and-the-constellation-of-orion.

37. Cindy Blankenship, Leaf Group, "Personalities of the Six Major Hawaiian Islands," USA Today (website), updated January 30, 2018, http://traveltips.usatoday.com/personalities-six-major-hawaiian-islands-108788.html.

Chapter Seven—Farewell

38. Rita Nakashima Brock and Gabriella Lettini, *Soul Repair: Recovering from Moral Injury after War* (Boston: Beacon Press, 2013).

39. Marilynn Larkin, "Physician Burnout Takes a Toll on U.S. Patients," Reuters (website), January 17, 2018, https://www.reuters.com/article/us-health -physicians-burnout/physician-burnout-takes-a-toll-on-u-s-patients-idUSKBN1F621U.

40. Carol Peckham, "Medscape National Physician Burnout & Depression Report 2018," Medscape (website), January 17, 2018, https://www.medscape.com/ slideshow/2018-lifestyle-burnout-depression-6009235.

41. Pamela Wible, MD, "What I've Learned from 757 Doctor Suicides," Pamela Wible MD, America's Leading Voice for Ideal Medical Care (website), posted October 28, 2017, http://www.idealmedicalcare.org/ive-learned-547 -doctor-suicides/.

42. Ed Pilkington, "US Military Struggling to Stop Suicide Epidemic Among War Veterans," The Guardian (website), February 1, 2013, https://www.theguardian.com/world/2013/feb/01/us-military-suicide -epidemic-veteran.

43. "United States Military Veteran Suicide," Wikipedia, The Free Encyclopedia (website), accessed May 10, 2018, https://en.wikipedia.org/wiki/United_ States_military_veteran_suicide.

44. See note 26 above.

45. "7 Hawaiian Legends Not to Be Ignored," Huffpost (website), updated December 6, 2017, https://www.huffingtonpost.com/2013/09/10/hawaiian -legends_n_3898664.html.

46. Katie Young Yamanaka, "Pele, Goddess of Fire and Volcanoes," Hawaii. com (website), accessed May 10, 2018, https://www.hawaii.com/discover/ culture/pele/.

Appendix

Essentials for the Road to Mana Hike

1. Movement

47. K. S. Hall, K. D. Hoerster, W. S. Yancy Jr., "Traumatic Stress Disorder, Physical Activity, and Eating Behaviors," *Epidemiologic Reviews* 37, no. 1 (January 2015): 103–115, https://doi.org/10.1093/epirev/mxu011.

48. T. Archer, A. Fredriksson, E. Schütz, "Influence of Physical Exercise on Neuroimmunological Functioning and Health: Aging and Stress," *Neurotoxicity Research* 20, no. 1, Springer Link (website), (January 16, 2015): 69–83, https://link.springer.com/article/10.1007/s12640-010-9224-9.

49. James McKinney, MD. "The Health Benefits of Physical Activity and Cardiorespiratory Fitness," *BC Medical Journal* 58, no. 3, BC Medical Journal (website), (April 2016): 131–137, http://www.bcmj.org/articles/health -benefits-physical-activity-and-cardiorespiratory-fitness

2. Nutrition

50. Eva Selhub, MD, "Nutritional Psychiatry: Your Brain on Food," *Harvard Health Blog*, Harvard Health Publishing (website), Updated April 5, 2018, https://www.health.harvard.edu/blog/nutritional-psychiatry-your-brain -on-food-201511168626.

51. T. C. Campbell, "The China Study," T. Colin Campbell Center for Nutrition Studies (website), accessed May 10, 2018, https://nutritionstudies.org/the-china-study/.

52. "Health Benefits of Eating Well," NHS inform (website), accessed May 10, 2018, https://www.nhsinform.scot/healthy-living/food-and-nutrition/eating-well/health-benefits-of-eating-well.

3. Mindfulness/Meditation

53. G. A. Marlatt, "Buddhist Philosophy and the Treatment of Addictive Behavior," *Cognitive and Behavioral Practice* 9 no. 1 (December 2002): 44–50, https://www.sciencedirect.com/science/article/pii/S1077722902800396.

54. S. Guendelman, S. Medeiros, H. Rampes, "Mindfulness and Emotion Regulation: Insights from Neurobiological, Psychological, and Clinical Studies," *Front. Psycho.* 6, (website), (March 2017), https://doi.org/10.3389/fpsyg.2017.00220.

55. Jeena Cho, "6 Scientifically Proven Benefits of Mindfulness and Meditation," Forbes (website), July 14, 2016, https://www.forbes.com/sites/jeenacho/2016/07/14/10-scientifically-proven-benefits-of-mindfulness-and-meditation/#40eed81263ce.

4. Massage

56. "Massage Therapy," National Center for Complementary and Integrative Health (website), September 24, 2017, https://nccih.nih.gov/health/massage.

57. Tiffany Field, "Massage Therapy Research Review," *Complementary Therapies in Clinical Practice* 20, no. 4 (November 2014): 224, https://doi.org/10.1016/j.ctcp.2014.07.002.

5. Yoga

58. Sujit Chandratreya, "Yoga: An Evidence-Based Therapy," *Journal of Mid-Life Health* 2, no. 1 (January–June 2011): 3–4, https://www.ncbi.nlm.nih.gov/pmc/articles/PMC3156498/.

59. Catherine Woodyard, "Exploring the Therapeutic Effects of Yoga and Its Ability to Increase Quality of Life," *International Journal of Yoga* 4, no. 2 (September 27, 2011): 49–54, doi: 10.4103/0973-6131.85485.

60. A. Büssing, A. Michalsen, S. B. S. Khalsa, S. Telles, K. Sherman, "Effects of Yoga on Mental and Physical Health: A Short Summary of Reviews," *Evidence-Based Complementary and Alternative Medicine* 2012, no. 165410 (July 18, 2012): 1–7, http://dx.doi.org/10.1155/2012/165410.

Made in the USA
San Bernardino, CA
25 July 2019